MEDIEVAL
MEDICINE

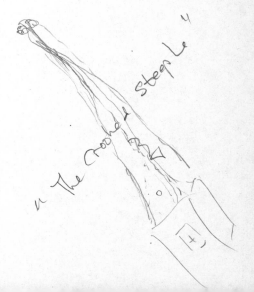

ABOUT THE AUTHOR

Toni Mount has been a history teacher for fifteen years. She has an MA by Research on medieval medical manuscripts from the University of Kent. Her previous books include *Everyday Life in Medieval London* and *The Medieval Housewife*. Her latest book, *A Year in the Life of Medieval Britain*, is due to be published this year by Amberley. Born in London, Toni now lives in Gravesend, Kent.

MEDIEVAL MEDICINE

ITS MYSTERIES AND SCIENCE

TONI MOUNT

AMBERLEY

To Glenn and all four generations of our family
– in sickness and in health

First published 2015
This edition published 2016

Amberley Publishing
The Hill, Stroud
Gloucestershire, GL5 4EP

www.amberley-books.com

Copyright © Toni Mount, 2015, 2016

The right of Toni Mount to be identified as
the Author of this work has been asserted
in accordance with the Copyrights, Designs
and Patents Act 1988.

ISBN 978 1 4456 5542 0 (paperback)
ISBN 978 1 4456 4410 3 (ebook)

British Library Cataloguing in Publication
Data.
A catalogue record for this book is
available from the British Library.

Typesetting and Origination by Amberley
Publishing.
Printed in the UK.

CONTENTS

CONTENTS

INTRODUCTION

Delighted as I was to be asked by Amberley to write a book on one of my pet subjects and my MA thesis – medieval medicine – I realised it was going to be difficult to keep the story within the bounds of some appropriate dates. Medical treatment in some form or another has its origins in prehistory and is still in development today, yet my remit was to extract and tell only the middle chapters of that never-ending quest for health.

The earliest remedies may have been taken instinctively by man, just as cats occasionally eat grass – something with no nutritional value for them – as an emetic or a laxative, perhaps to rid their gut of the inedible parts of their prey, fur, feathers and bones, or even the furballs accumulated from grooming.[1] Elephants actively seek out mineral 'licks', soils that contain vital elements otherwise lacking in their diets.[2] It is more than likely that prehistoric man had similar behaviours, eating certain plants that made him feel better, eased his headache or settled his queasy stomach. Willow bark was discovered in a Neanderthal burial site in Iraq, dated to 60,000 years BC.[3] We know that Ötzi the Iceman, a mummy from 5,000 years ago found in 1991 by two German tourists in the mountains of western Austria, carried in his pack an edible mushroom that was used as a laxative.[4] So where to begin the story and where to end it?

I decided to begin by looking at the origins of the diseases themselves. Most have evolved from the ailments suffered by other animal and bird species, a process that continues with the advent of Ebola. The natural host species for Ebola was believed to be primates, but a recent discovery suggests it may be bats.[5] Man the hunter-gatherer was generally healthier than man the farmer for three reasons. Firstly, as a hunter, his contact with animals was limited to pursuing, killing and eating them. As a farmer, he lived close to his domesticated livestock, giving their diseases far greater opportunity to make the species jump. Secondly, as a wanderer, the hunter constantly moved on before the local environment became too contaminated with his waste, but the farmer stayed put, making sewage disposal a problem and raising the possibility of his flocks fouling the water supply. Finally, with human populations increasing and living in larger communities, diseases could develop and spread, becoming both endemic and, occasionally, epidemic – something that just couldn't happen in the small, mobile family units of the hunter-gatherers. For the stay-at-home farmers, medicine became evermore important and necessary.

The practice of religion and medicine often went hand in hand in early societies and the split between the two happened slowly and reluctantly. By medieval times, the Church was still closely associated with both the training and the conduct of medicine, in practice and theory, but what effect did Christianity have on the ideas and means of treatment?

Then there are the mysteries of diagnosis and prognosis, some of which date back to Ancient Greece, while others are still used in doctors' surgeries today. Along the way, this book looks at some of the weird and wonderful remedies – weird because they involved magic charms and strange ingredients, from half a mouse to the blood of a dragon, and wonderful because some of them actually worked – from the antiseptic spiders' webs to the painkilling willow-tree bark and meadowsweet plant. Medieval doctors used other herbs and even animal products, such as snail slime, which only recently have been found to do what was claimed.

Medieval medicine involved other 'sciences' too: astronomy, astrology, alchemy and foretelling the future. All were vital to ensure the correct method was used in treating the patient. This book examines how and why such knowledge was important, how dealing with and tending the wounded on the battlefield advanced medical treatment and anatomy and why progress was often a case of two steps forward and one step back.

The part played by women, whether as the doctor or patient, is explored. How did they deal with pregnancy, contraception and childbirth and what was the role of midwives in medieval forensics? The legal side of medicine was as much in evidence then as now, with cases of malpractice, negligence and the pursuit of unpaid fees being taken to court. Medical practitioners were expected to be upright, moral pillars of the community, but that wasn't always the way things worked out.

At times progress seems to have been nonexistent, with a reliance on ancient textbooks continuing into the early nineteenth century when some aspects of medieval medicine were still being taught and practised. For this reason, knowing where to end this book was as hard as knowing where to begin. Medicine was a field of knowledge full of anomalies, conundrums and riddles and although modern research has managed to unravel some of the mysteries, for every puzzle worked out another seems to take its place.

I hope this book opens up some of these intriguing questions for modern readers, but many of the medical detective stories have yet to be solved. Modern science still doesn't have all the answers. Although it has now been confirmed that the Black Death was definitely bubonic plague, this doesn't explain some of the characteristics of the medieval epidemic, so these matters still need explaining. Sometimes, we literally don't know 'whodunnit'. This is the case with the 'sweating sickness' which raged across England just as the first Tudor monarch began his reign in 1485, only to disappear just as mysteriously in the mid-sixteenth century. Recent research may have nailed the culprit, but the jury has yet to pass judgement.

This book tells the unfinished story of medicine even as some of its medieval practices are currently being revived in man's continuing quest to conquer disease. Leeches are making a comeback in microsurgery and honey is being 'rediscovered' as an effective antibiotic and promoter of healing mechanisms. As the mysteries of medieval medicine continue to be re-examined, who can tell what other strange methods of treatment or unlikely sounding ingredients may prove to be the next wonders of medicine?

Toni Mount
December 2014

I

DIRT, DISEASE AND DANGER

> The lane called Ebbegate used to be a right of way until ...
> Thomas at Wytte and William de Hockele built latrines which
> stuck out from the walls of the houses from [which] human
> filth falls out onto the heads of passers-by.
>
> Evidence from a London court case, 1321

Imagine how revolting that must have been for those unfortunate
passers-by, showered in poo while going about their daily work.
More importantly, think of the hazard to their health and
well-being. Surprisingly, though, the situation that brought about
the court case quoted above was a prosecution for nuisance: the
inconvenience of people being doused in the latrine contents as
they walked beneath in Ebbegate Lane. Despite living in such
unhygienic conditions in the crowded streets of fourteenth-century
London, the idea that this was a serious health risk was hardly
considered, unless the stink became overwhelming.

Medieval folk generally agreed – physicians and scholars among
them – that diseases arose from bad smells, foul airs or 'miasmas',
as the later Tudors called them. This often meant that they got it
right; effluent discharged from latrines, piles of animal dung in
the street, discarded offal from the butchers or fishmongers and

stagnant water all smelled bad and could well give rise to disease. Miles Robinson, a butcher in the city of York, was ordered by the authority of Davygate ward to remove 'all that great dunghill' in his yard because it was 'most perilous for infecting the aire'.[1] Every so often the authorities in towns and cities would have a purge of street cleaning, usually when a disease was already afflicting the population or an important visitor, such as the king, was expected. But if the smell wasn't too bad or the prevailing wind blew the pong away, the refuse was often left to accumulate until it became such an obstruction that it was worth the authorities' expense to pay someone to remove it, or to pass a new by-law to force local residents to clear it away.

As far as it went, the miasma theory seemed to fit the facts – that nasty smells gave rise to disease and the unpleasant breath of a sick person carried his contagion and might infect others. Early medical books lumped together 'fevers, pestilence and poisons' as all emanating from foul airs. Now that we understand more about how bacteria and viruses are spread and multiply, it is easy to see that these ideas seemed sensible at the time. For example, by law a leper must not stand upwind of a healthy person when speaking to them for fear the wind would carry his contagious breath and transfer the disease. No one realised then that leprosy is, in fact, difficult to catch and never by airborne infection. However, in the case of coughs, colds and many other illnesses, these seemed to prove the miasma theory.

How Did Diseases Originate?

In order to survive, diseases need a host population of a critical size and density; without this, once everyone had contracted the illness and either died or developed immunity and recovered there would be nobody left to infect and the disease itself would die out. For these reasons, early man as a hunter-gatherer, living in small nomadic groups, would have suffered from very few

infectious diseases. His mixed diet of meat, vegetables and fruit
was a healthy one and he got – of necessity – plenty of exercise
in catching or collecting his food. However, wild animals, living
in large flocks or herds, did suffer from endemic diseases. Only
when man settled down in permanent communities, alongside
his domesticated livestock, did certain diseases make the 'species
jump', mutating and infecting man. (Modern research has shown
that most contagious diseases afflicting humans have originated
from some other animal or bird – the influenza pandemic of
1918–19, which killed more people than the First World War,
is an example and is thought to have originated in the pigs
brought in to feed the troops.) Not only were new infections
evolving among the farmers but man's new diet, containing a lot
of cereals and less variety otherwise, wasn't so nutritious, lacking
in iron, which led to a high proportion of these more sedentary
populations suffering from anaemia. This lack of iron in the blood
could cause lethargy, slower rates of healing and lower resistance
to other pathogens.[2]

Returning to historical sources, what diseases did mankind suffer
from in the past? There is a description of an illness that sounds
similar to chicken pox (varicella) recorded over 2,000 years ago in
ancient Babylonia. Historians think that the Anglo-Saxon ailment
of 'watery-elf' disease was actually chicken pox.[3] The treatment
for it at the time consisted of mixing 'English herbs' with holy
water and singing these words repeatedly over the patient while
he drank the herbal remedy: 'May the Earth destroy thee with
all her might.' The Anglo-Saxon doctor, or 'leech' as they called
him, was trying to drive out the evil spirit that was making the
patient unwell. In this case, they were mixing herbal lore, magical
charms, myths and religious ideas just to make sure the patient
had every advantage. In the late ninth and early tenth century AD,
the Persian philosopher Muhammad ibn Zakariya Razi (known as
Rhazes in the West) wrote down the first definitive information on

chicken pox, but up until the sixteenth century it was still being thought of as a milder form of smallpox.

In AD 910, Rhazes also wrote *A Treatise on the Smallpox and Measles*, a work that was later translated from Arabic into Latin for Western scholars. In the treatise, he distinguished between these two highly infectious diseases, which were often confused in the early stages of the illness with chicken pox and rubella (German measles), as they all caused skin rashes. The medieval term 'spotted fever' covered all these diseases, as well as scarlet fever, hives and any other ailment that produced a rash and a raised temperature. If it was difficult for physicians of the day to tell one from another, the problem is much greater for us today, working from their descriptions of the symptoms. Rhazes suggested that measles (rubeola) was 'more to be dreaded than smallpox' (variola). He thought that a person's basic constitution determined whether he suffered from smallpox or measles:

Bodies that are lean, bilious, hot and dry are more disposed to the measles than to the smallpox.

The early origins of the measles virus are currently an interesting source of scholarly disagreement. In 2007, Dr Mary Dobson wrote that '[measles] may have evolved from the canine distemper of dogs or the bovine rinderpest of cattle several thousand years ago [and] probably spread out from its original urban hearth in Mesopotamia around 3000 BC'.[4] It is clear that Rhazes was also familiar with a disease he called 'measles', but recent research has cast some doubt as to exactly what ailment he was describing. In 2010, Japanese researchers reported on their studies into the genetics of the measles virus and discovered that it evolved from the rinderpest virus, a cattle pathogen, as recently as the eleventh or twelfth century AD.[5] So what was Rhazes referring to in his treatise? Has measles evolved as a human disease more than once?

We are left with the intriguing question: could King Alfred the Great (AD 849–899) and his contemporaries ever have caught the measles or not?

Mumps (parotitis) was described in the writings of Hippocrates around 400 BC, as was a sickness that may have been scarlet fever, in this latter case referring to the patient's sore throat and skin ulcers. Diphtheria is another disease with a long history and there are references to it in ancient Syria and Egypt. Again, the first clinical description of diphtheria appears in the works of Hippocrates.

One infectious disease that doesn't seem to have an ancient history is whooping cough or pertussis. The first definite mention of this horrible ailment is of an outbreak in Paris in 1414, although the reference is found in Moulton's *The Mirror of Health*, which wasn't published until 1640. Before there was any medical understanding of bacteria, pertussis was believed to be caused, possibly, by physical contact with – or the miasma given off by – dying flowers, particularly orchids. As their petals began to turn black, it was thought to be a sign of the inevitable onset of the '100-day cough' for any child close by. At whatever date this disease first afflicted humans, various weird treatments and 'cures' were quickly invented, all of which sound more like witches' spells than medicinal remedies:

Take a caterpillar, wrap it in a small bag of muslin, and hang the bag around the neck of the affected child. The caterpillar will die and the child will be cured. Or pour a bowl of milk and get a ferret to lap from the bowl. After the child drinks the rest of the milk, she will recover.

Woodlice mixed with breast milk, a broth made from snails, the hoot of an owl, breathing in the scent of cattle, sheep or horses, even passing the child over and under a donkey – preferably one which was braying – were alternative cures for whooping cough which date to the Tudor period.[6]

The Plague

The words 'plague' or 'Black Death' send shivers down our spines even today. Although the chances of catching the plague are minimal in Western society (there are up to twenty cases in the USA each year[7]), modern medicine can treat it effectively with antibiotics and the chances of dying from it are very low, it is as if we have inherited a fear and loathing of the disease so dreaded by our medieval ancestors. The disease had many names at the time: the Great Mortality, the pestilence, the Great Plague or even the pox. The popular term 'the Black Death' wasn't current at the time, despite being so appropriate – it was coined by the British historian Elizabeth Penrose in 1823 – but this is how one of its victims, a Welsh poet named Jeuan Gethin, managed to describe the disease before he died of it in 1349:

We see death coming into our midst like black smoke, a plague that cuts off the young, a rootless phantom that has no mercy for fair countenance. Woe is me of the shilling (bubo) in the armpit; it is seething, terrible, where ever it may come, a head that gives pain and causes a loud cry, a burden carried under the arms, a painful angry knob, a white lump.

Although this medieval scourge seemed to be an entirely new sickness when it began its deadly work in the mid-fourteenth century, the Bible refers to 'a pestilence' being sent by God upon the people of Egypt, in Exodus 10:15. Might this have been the first known instance of *the* plague? And in Samuel I, in about 1320 BC, the Philistines stole the Ark of the Covenant from the Israelites and returned home:

The Lord's hand was heavy upon the people of Ashod and
its vicinity; He brought devastation upon them and afflicted
them with tumours. And rats appeared in their land, and
death and destruction were throughout the city … He afflicted
the people of the city, both young and old, with an outbreak
of tumours in the groin.

The Anglo-Saxon monk known as the Venerable Bede wrote
about what he called 'the Plague of Justinian' that swept through
Europe in the sixth and seventh centuries AD. In his *De gestis
Anglorum*, he records that in the time of Vortigern, King of the
Britons, not enough people were left alive to carry the dead to their
graves. The plague had raced westwards from Constantinople,
which was under attack from followers of the new religion of
Islam, brought from Arabia, via Egypt, along with the teachings
of the prophet Mohammed. In Constantinople, at the peak
of the epidemic, up to 10,000 people a day were said to have
died. The disease ravaged and perhaps even fatally weakened
Justinian's Roman Empire and moved on across Europe to
England, where it was also known as the Plague of Cadwalader's
Time, then crossing to Ireland, which it laid waste in 664. The
described symptom of swellings in the neck, armpit or groin,
called 'buboes', is characteristic of bubonic plague. These buboes
– from the Greek *boubon*, meaning 'swollen groin' – were caused
when the lymph glands closest to the site of the infected fleabite
became engorged with white blood cells as the body tried to fight
off the contagion. But *bubo* in Latin means 'owl', a creature of
darkness, and owls were sometimes used to decorate the margins
of medieval plague treatises.

That the Black Death was bubonic plague, caused by the bites
of infected rat fleas, was commonly accepted for many years but,
quite recently, there was some doubt about it. Bubonic plague
is endemic to certain areas of the world; those that have been

identified with reasonable certainty are Uganda, western Arabia, Kurdistan, northern India, China and the Gobi Desert and the western states of the USA. The plague bacterium, *Yersinia pestis,* may live for years in its rodent host population of black rats, prairie dogs, marmots, chipmunks, ground squirrels or rabbits. It can survive in the soil of their burrows without affecting the animals. Then, from time to time, it erupts in the form of minor, localised epidemics and may pass into the human population through infected fleas deserting the dead rodent hosts in search of fresh blood. Typically, dead rodents are found lying around in considerable numbers, so the fleas cannot find another living rodent host.

Unlike the Black Death or influenza, modern bubonic plague moves slowly. It is not contagious from person to person, except in its pneumonic form, which affects the lungs and can be passed on in airborne droplets by coughing. This hardly fits the profile of the medieval pandemic which spread like fire in a haystack and definitely seems to have been passed rapidly from one to another among the people. Neither do piles of dead rats feature in the descriptions of the time, which surely couldn't have gone unnoticed – if they existed. For these reasons, some scholars have recently argued that, instead of bubonic plague, anthrax or a highly contagious haemorrhagic fever – something like the Ebola virus – might be possible alternative causes of the infamous Black Death.

Since the 1990s, archaeologists across Europe have been excavating burial sites and cemeteries dating to the times of plague. This is a hazardous procedure because the pathogens that cause the disease may still be viable and precautions have to be taken to protect those involved in the dig, the storage and the laboratory analysis of any specimens retrieved, as well as the rest of the population who could be at risk if any pathogen escaped. DNA analysis was carried out by a team of researchers at Oxford University's Ancient Biomolecules Centre on the remains of sixty-one plague victims from across Europe and found *no trace of* Yersinia *DNA*.

Forensic paleopathology (the study of ancient diseases) has moved on rapidly and more recent techniques in obtaining DNA from sources that are centuries old, along with new and more accurate analysis of the samples, seem to have unravelled the mystery. Experts have been able to extract and analyse DNA from the pulp found inside the teeth of skeletons exhumed from sites like the East Smithfield plague cemetery in London. Once a disease pathogen – whether a bacterium or virus – gets into the victim's bloodstream, its DNA is found throughout the body tissues until the patient recovers. Even then, the victim's tissues may contain antibodies to the disease. Since these victims never recovered, the pathogenic DNA is likely to be present – if it has survived the centuries of burial. The analysis done in 2010–11 of samples taken from twenty-seven sites in five European countries have shown that *Yersinia pestis* was indeed the agent of death.[9] It also proves that all the precautions taken were necessary, since we know this bacterium can survive for years in the soil. Evidence of other pathogens analysed by a French team from a plague cemetery in Venice in 2012 included anthrax, typhus, typhoid fever, smallpox, louse-borne trench fever and louse-borne relapsing fever as well as plague.[10]

Having answered the question as to the cause of the plague, more questions have been raised by the new discoveries. Having proved that the Black Death was definitely the bubonic plague, new explanations are needed as to why it was so contagious and lethal in the medieval period compared to today. Was it an especially virulent strain of the bacterium? Further research has shown that it wasn't very different from the modern strain and no more contagious, so scientists have looked instead at the vectors of the disease, the means by which it is transferred from one victim to the next. Rat fleas have always been presumed guilty ever since rats were proven to be the most common source of the plague, but rat fleas only attempt to feed on humans once there are no rodents available. As we've seen, dead rats don't seem to have been a feature of the medieval plague epidemics. The presence of louse-borne trench fever and louse-borne relapsing fever in those Venetian victims may be a clue. New theories are currently being tested as to whether the human flea and the human louse could be the carriers once the plague has entered the human population from the rat.[11] If that had happened, rats and their fleas would no longer feature in the cycle of contagion and the disease would be passed on by these human parasites, from one victim to the next, in the time it takes a flea to jump or a louse to transfer. How long does it take for an infestation of headlice to afflict a whole class of primary school children these days?

However, there are still unanswered questions, in particular the incubation period of the disease. This is the time when a victim has already caught the infection and the bacteria are multiplying inside him, but he has no symptoms, as yet, and feels fine. He goes about his work, spreading the infection to those he meets until, finally, he falls ill and has to take to his bed. Bubonic plague has an incubation period of only a few days – not much time to travel very far or to spread the contagion to many people. This was one of the arguments in favour of the Black Death being some form of viral haemorrhagic fever which, typically, have incubation periods of about thirty days – plenty of time for ships to carry the infection from port to port or for travellers to make long journeys and meet countless possible new victims.

This longer incubation period seems to have been borne out in the historical records. The Black Death arrived in Sicily early in October 1347, aboard a flotilla of Genoese galleys that brought the infection into the port of Messina from the Crimea according to the chronicler Michael of Piazza. Strangely, the Italian chronicler talks of the crews as having 'sickness clinging to their very bones', but actually says that the men were displaying no symptoms. Were they simply unfortunate enough to arrive as the plague was first noticed in the city? Whatever the case, within a few days the plague had taken a firm grip on the city. These Genoese sailors could be important in identifying the cause of the Black Death – with a long incubation period, they could not be to blame for its immediate appearance in Messina upon their arrival; with a short period, they would have been ill already when they reached the port. Also, the authorities set up quarantine measures – the Italian word means 'forty' – and forty days of isolation for incomers would hardly be necessary if the plague symptoms appeared within just a few days.

With it already too late to save themselves, the citizens of Messina turned on the mariners they thought had brought them this terrifying cargo and drove them from the port, thus sending the disease around the Mediterranean. With hundreds of victims dying every day and the slightest contact with the sick seeming to guarantee rapid infection, the population panicked. The few officials who might have organised some measures to mitigate the danger were themselves among the first to die. The people fled from their doomed city into the fields and vineyards of southern Sicily, seeking safety in isolation and carrying the plague with them through the countryside.

By June 1348 the plague was in Paris, but the fear of it and the horror stories travelled even faster. Towns and villages as yet unaffected could only wait and pray, regarding every stranger, however healthy they appeared, with deep suspicion as the possible carrier of the deadly contagion. Again, this would suggest a long incubation period. However, not all cities were devastated as Messina. Milan was spared, as was Liege (now in Belgium), the Bearn region in the Pyrenees and much of the eastern parts of the German states. But at least a third and maybe half of western Europe's population would die in 'the Pestilence'. This meant that around twenty to thirty million people died of the plague between

1347 and 1350 out of a population of around sixty million. As a comparison, the so-called Spanish flu epidemic of 1918 possibly killed fifty million worldwide, but the mortality rate in proportion to the total population was obviously relatively small compared to the impact of the plague.

This great social and medical catastrophe hit England as hard as any other country in 1348–49, and because of the rich documentary evidence surviving from fourteenth-century England we can study both the personal and social impact of the disease. Up to 1300, the population of England and Wales had increased dramatically to around six million. Unusually warm weather and soft rains had produced year after year of bumper harvests and, like the crops, mankind had flourished. But the second decade of the fourteenth century saw bad weather, poor harvests and famine throughout Europe, insufficient food for the much expanded population. So when the pestilence arrived, it found mankind an easy, undernourished target. Was this why it proved so virulent and claimed the lives of such a high proportion of its victims?

The medicine of the fourteenth century was capable of some great achievements – limbs could be successfully amputated, wounds cauterised, stitched and treated with antiseptic applications, herbal remedies could cure minor ailments like headaches and upset stomachs – but in the face of the pestilence it was helpless. Contemporary English medical texts and chronicles played down their descriptions of reactions to the plague and its particular symptoms, unlike their Continental counterparts who distinguished it from other epidemics by its speed, severity and widespread nature. The English *Brut Chronicle* wrote in despair, 'In these days was death without sorrow, wedding without friendship, wilful penance, and dearth without scarcity, and fleeing without refuge or succour.'

The English chronicler Geoffrey le Baker noted that recovery was more likely if buboes developed than if the discoloured carbuncles – known as God's tokens and signifying the end was nigh – appeared all over the body, especially on the chest. The buboes might blacken, suppurate and give off a vile stench. They usually appeared within two or three days, but were not always present. In his writing on the plague, the English physician John of Arderne explained that just as an owl (*bubo* in Latin) loved the dark, secluded places, so the buboes appeared in those of the body – the armpit or the groin. The aggressive owl in the margin of surgeon John Bradmore's *Philomena* marks the appropriate section of his text on the plague. Bradmore's work, written in the fifteenth century, reveals – as do many other English works – a reliance on the writings of Continental authors as regards the cause, prevention and treatment of the disease. Particularly popular were the works of Guy de Chauliac, surgeon to Pope Clement VI at Avignon, who had witnessed the plague's devastation there in 1348, and those of John of Burgundy, whose tract on the plague, written in 1365 and soon translated into English, had a wide circulation in England. By the time of Bradmore, the fact that the plague kept returning was well understood: England suffered badly in 1361, 1368–69, 1371, 1375, 1390, 1400 and 1405. The plague pandemic of 1348 had become endemic and was here to stay until the late seventeenth century.

We have a contemporary account known as the *Historia Roffensis*, the chronicle of the cathedral priory of Rochester in Kent, dated from 1314 to 1350. It is believed to have been written by William Dene and is now in the British Library:

As a result [of the Great Mortality] there was such a shortage of servants, craftsmen and workmen, and of agricultural workers and labourers ... Alas, this mortality devoured such a multitude of both sexes that no one could be found to carry the bodies of the dead to burial, but men and women carried the bodies of their own little ones to church on their shoulders and threw them into the mass graves ... From his modest household the Bishop of Rochester [Hamo de Hythe] lost 4 priests, 5 squires, 10 household servants, 7 young clerks and 6 pages, leaving no one in any office to serve him. At Malling [in Kent] he appointed two abbesses who promptly died. No one remained alive there except 4 professed nuns and 4 novices, and the bishop committed the custody of the temporalities to one of them and the spiritualities to another, since no adequate person could be found to fill the post of abbess.

This means Bishop Hamo had one nun carry out the spiritual duties of the abbess and put another in charge of the secular side of the business. Incidentally, Hamo was old and frail yet survived the visitation of the Black Death unscathed.

Most Continental scholars at the time believed the plague originated in a universal pollution of the air, brought about by a deadly planetary conjunction of Mars, Saturn and Jupiter in Aquarius. This caused corrupted vapours to be released from the earth, spreading the poisonous air or miasma. This explained its widespread transmission and contagion, which came about through three forms of contact: via the pores of the skin, via respiration or via the gaze of an infected person. Flight was reckoned the best course of action, but the authors of plague tracts also suggested preventive measures, such as quarantine for all incomers and their goods and, to a lesser extent, cures. Regarding the avoidance of pestilential air, one should live in 'correcting or purifying air, avoiding contact with infectious persons'. The use of sweet-smelling aromatics was another preventive – marjoram, savoury and mint for the poor; wood of aloes, amber and musk for the rich – to counter the stink of putrefaction and corruption, not only for individuals at home, but strewn in the streets too. Renewed legislation on sanitation was issued by many civic authorities in England in the years following the plague, from better drainage and orders against offal and manure in the streets to the attempted removal of whole communities from town centres. People like tanners and dyers and fishmongers whose trades created bad smells – stinks being one and the same as those poisonous miasmas – were encouraged, sometimes ordered, to leave town, at least temporarily. However, there was an alternative view held by some that people working in those smelly trades had an immunity to the plague, so they spent long hours attempting to acquire the same by inhaling the stench of the public latrines or sitting by sewers; folk were that desperate, they would try anything.

Diet was reckoned important in avoiding the plague; it should be light, but without fruit or any food cooked in honey. Vinegar could be mixed with just about everything and garlic was especially effective. Moderate exercise was advised, but no hot baths because they would open the pores of the skin to the miasma of contagion. Keeping the body purged and cleansed was all-important, and regular bloodletting was recommended. Medications such as Armenian bolus, Lemnian earth and agaric as simples, and compounds containing theriac, emeralds, pills of aloes, saffron and myrrh were recommended for their cleansing and invigorating properties or as antidotes to the poison. Ultimately, everyone was advised to think of their soul and do whatever they could to appease God's divine anger at the sins of men.

These medical, social and psychological measures show how doctors' opinions were taken into account regarding the civic and community efforts made in an attempt to lessen the dreadful impact of the plague. Just how effective these medical ideas might have been is difficult to assess. Many people must have felt, as a contemporary English poem stated, that 'against death is worth no medicine'.

By the fifteenth century, recurrences of plague were met with the same basic measures that had been used in 1348 and again in the 1360s. The plague came to be regarded as just another of the lethal cocktail of epidemic diseases that were part of English life and included typhus, smallpox, epidemic dysentery (the summer flux), malaria (in East Anglia and the Thames-side marshes of Kent and Essex) and, later, the mysterious 'sweating sickness'. In England, a manuscript on plague that was circulating around 1480 was thought to be so important that it was among the first books to be printed on an English press. It was reprinted in 1536 and became a standard textbook of its time for the avoidance, prevention and treatment of the pestilence. The author describes himself as the Bishop of Aarhus in Denmark and claims to have practised physic (medicine) at the University of Montpellier, which specialised in training medical doctors. He describes his preventive measures:

> [In the time of the pestilence] I might not eschew the company of people for I went from house to house, because of my poverty, to cure sick folk. Therefore bread or a sponge sopped in vinegar I took with me, holding it to my mouth and nose, because all sour things stopped the ways of humours and suffereth no venomous thing to enter into a man's body; and so I escaped the pestilence, my fellows supposing I should not live. These foresaid things I have proved by myself.

An interesting point here is that the sponge soaked in vinegar may have been an effective way of preventing a disease that was passed by airborne droplet infection. But the author raises another question which has yet to be answered:

> Wherefore one dieth and another dieth not, in a town when men be dead in one house and in another house there dieth none.

It seems there is still much to learn about the plague that devastated Europe centuries ago. The research goes on ...

Leprosy

Leprosy, or Hanson's disease as it was renamed in the twentieth century, was as much a social disease as a physical one in medieval times and continued to be so. This chronic bacterial infection was given its new name in an effort to remove the stigma attached to it. Mentioned in the Bible, it was an ancient disease, but medieval people believed it was caused by lechery and immoral sex and was the outward physical evidence of a corrupt soul. Hence, lepers were to be shunned not only because of their contagious sickness, but also because they were sinful. Folk believed that lecherous men and women, especially those who were vain about their beautiful looks, were all too likely to be afflicted with leprosy as a divine punishment. The poet Robert Henryson, writing in the fifteenth century, added a kind of postscript to the story of Troilus and Cressida as told by other writers, such as Geoffrey Chaucer in his *Troilus and Criseyde*. In Henryson's version, the beautiful but flawed heroine, Cresseid, ended up in a leper house with 'my greit mischief quhilk na man can amend' (my terrible disease which nobody can cure), even her lovely singing voice reduced to a harsh croak, and all because she was wanton, having fallen in love with the Greek Diomede despite having declared her undying love for the Trojan Troilus, as well as vain and proud.[12] It was even believed that a child could be born with leprosy if it was conceived during the mother's menstruation – a time when she was supposed to refrain from having sex, according to Church law.[13]

Clearly, people had no idea of the true cause of leprosy, but they reckoned it was extremely contagious. This is another medical mystery because leprosy is one of the least contagious of bacterial infections. One reason why this was believed may be that other skin problems could have been mistaken for the early symptoms of leprosy. This seems to have been the case for the unfortunate widow Joanna Nightingale, who was treated as a leper by her family and neighbours in Brentford, London, but didn't have the disease after all (see chapter 4).

Archaeological evidence from medieval cemeteries has proved that, in Britain, leprosy dates back to at least the fourth century AD. Skeletons have been found that show the unmistakeable (to modern science) ravages of the disease in the bones. The symptoms, which may take years to show themselves, consist of nodules on the skin that eventually cause permanent internal damage to the bones, especially at the extremities, where nerve damage causes numbness of the tissues, so the patient is unaware of injury. Further disfigurement may occur around the eyes, nose, lips and ears.

Founding or giving money or charitable donations to leper hospitals was a good way to earn time off purgatory, so they thought. The Church ruled that lepers had to be isolated for fear of corrupting healthy and morally upright folk, and between AD 1100 and Henry VIII's destruction of the monasteries around 1540 anywhere from three hundred to five hundred of these 'lazar houses' were set up in England and run by monks or nuns. Many didn't last very long because leprosy was actually on the wane in Europe from about 1300; this is another riddle still to be solved. Some lazar houses became more general hospitals, treating other diseases; some were converted to 'pest houses' for plague victims or places of quarantine; others simply fell into decay. Yet the lepers themselves were a conundrum. Sinful and immoral they may have been, but the Church saw them as already suffering and paying for their sins in this life, instead of waiting until after death, as everyone else would do in that mysterious place, purgatory. This meant that lepers were already on their way to redemption, so their prayers carried more weight than most with the heavenly authorities. To aid a leper, give him charity and ask him to pray for you in return was, therefore, an excellent, Christian thing to do to benefit your own soul.

The Sweating Sickness

This is yet another disease with mysteries of its own and, as with the plague, modern research raises questions as to its cause. During the twentieth century, it was generally thought that the 'sweating sickness' or *sudor Anglicus* – the English sweat – was probably another acute form of viral infection, possibly a virulent form of the flu. But some of the symptoms and the profile of the sickness just didn't fit with those of influenza. Influenza epidemics occur in cold weather and mortality is highest among the elderly, whereas epidemics of the sweat happened in the summer and early autumn and tended to claim the lives of otherwise fit and healthy young adults. Henry VIII's second wife, Anne Boleyn, is believed to have contracted the sweat and survived, but her near-contemporary Henry Brandon, Duke of Suffolk, did not, succumbing during the epidemic of 1551.

There were six epidemics of the sweat, in 1485, 1506, 1517, 1528, 1551 and 1578. They were confined to England, except in 1528–29, when it spread to Europe. Apart from the outbreak in 1506, which was quite mild, the epidemics had a very high mortality rate. The Tudor physician John Caius, who blamed 'dirt and filth' for this disease, was practising in Shrewsbury in 1551 when an outbreak occurred. He described the progress of the disease in his *A Boke or Counseill Against the Disease Commonly Called the Sweate, or Sweatyng Sicknesse,* printed in 1552. According to Caius, the illness began with a headache, giddiness and lethargy. After a few hours, drenching sweats began and were accompanied by severe headache, delirium, breathlessness and a rapid pulse. Death could happen within two to eighteen hours after the first symptoms. Caius tells us, 'Some [died] within two hours, some merry at dinner and dead at supper.'

If the patient survived for twenty-four hours, they would usually make a complete recovery. Unfortunately, having recovered, as with flu, the patient had no immunity from any future attack. Each epidemic was short-lived, lasting for just a few weeks.

Recently, Drs Vanya Gant and Guy Thwaites of St Thomas' Hospital in London think they may have identified *sudor Anglicus* as an early version of a disease called hantavirus pulmonary syndrome, which made headlines in the summer of 1993 in the south-western USA. According to Gant, the 'similarities between the two are striking':

First, there is hanta's rapid course. Basically, you've got a headache in the morning, you're short of breath in the afternoon, you take to your bed at teatime, and you're on a respirator by midnight. Second, sweating sickness left its victims breathless. Hanta also leaves people gasping, filling their lungs with fluid.[14]

Hantavirus is endemic in certain species of rapidly breeding rodents – in the USA it was the deer mouse – and becomes active towards the end of the summer when the rodent population is at its maximum. And just as the sweating sickness did, hantavirus also kills robust adults. Gant and Thwaites say that if they could exhume the remains of the Duke of Suffolk from his resting place they might determine the DNA identity of the sweating sickness, but there are no plans to disturb his grave at present. Perhaps one medieval medical mystery has been solved.

How a Splinter Could Be Fatal

Before the discovery of antibiotics, a splinter in the finger – such a minor matter today – could prove fatal. A wound, though small, could become infected with the bacteria that cause tetanus (*Clostridium tetani*). Today this happens rarely because in the West most babies are vaccinated against it, but in medieval times tetanus was a very real possibility if a wound came into contact with soil, manure or even house dust. Agricultural labourers and those who worked with animals must have been especially vulnerable and their number would have included the majority of the population. If a wound did get infected, the symptoms were muscle stiffness, which developed into muscle spasms that clenched the jaw – hence its other name, lockjaw – and swallowing becoming increasingly difficult. Tetanus bacteria produce neurotoxins which eventually cause paralysis – the patient can no longer breathe and death results. Nowadays, if a patient does become infected with tetanus, it can be treated with antibiotics, muscle relaxants and, if necessary, they can be put on a ventilator to keep them breathing until the infection subsides, but back then no such treatments were dreamed of.

Blood poisoning, or septicaemia/sepsis, was common – so common, in fact, that it was called 'wound fever' and anyone unlucky enough to suffer an injury in which the skin was broken almost expected to suffer an infection as a matter of course. Even today, the National Health Service in the United Kingdom reckons that more than 100,000 people are taken into hospital suffering from sepsis every year and as many as 37,000 will die from the resulting complications, despite modern medical intervention and antibiotics. Without hygiene or any knowledge of antiseptics, you can imagine that such deaths were not infrequent:

> In sepsis, the body's immune system goes into overdrive, setting off … widespread inflammation, swelling and blood clotting. This can lead to a significant decrease in blood pressure, which can mean the blood supply to vital organs such as the brain, heart and kidneys is reduced. If not treated quickly, sepsis can eventually lead to multiple organ failure and death.[15]

Early symptoms of sepsis usually develop quickly and can include a high fever, shivering and chills with a rapid pulse and breathing.

Battlefield injuries could often result in these serious infections, as we will see in chapter 9, but there are numerous records of sudden deaths by accident.

Royal Accidents

The Scottish royal line seems to have been spectacularly accident-prone: Alexander III, King of Scots, died in a fall from his horse in the dark while riding to visit the queen at Kinghorn in Fife on 18 March 1286 because it was her birthday the next day. He had spent the evening at Edinburgh Castle celebrating and was advised not to ride to Fife because the weather was terrible and it was late at night. Alexander went anyway and became separated from his guides. It was assumed that his horse lost its footing in the dark. The forty-four-year-old king was found dead on the shore the following morning with a broken neck. Some sources say that he fell off a cliff, but apparently there is no cliff at the site where his body was found, just a steep, rocky embankment that nonetheless would have been enough to prove fatal in a fall in the dark.

Another Scottish royal casualty was James II, who had a large number of cannon imported from Flanders for the siege of Roxburgh Castle in 1460. Fascinated by his new weapons of war, James was attempting to fire one of these cannon when it exploded and killed him. A contemporary source tells us, 'As the King stood near a piece of artillery, his thigh bone was dug in two with a piece of misframed gun that brake in shooting, by which he was stricken to the ground and died hastily.'[16]

A third untimely royal accident ended in the death of Alexander Stewart, Duke of Albany and brother to the next King of Scots, James III. The unfortunate duke was killed – one source says 'as a spectator' – at a tournament in Paris on 7 August 1485, when a flying splinter from the shattered lance of one of the contestants pierced his eye and entered his brain. Had Alexander been one of the competitors taking part in the joust he should have been wearing a visor to protect his face, so it seems quite possible that he was either just a very unlucky spectator or an extremely careless contestant. So that was yet another fatal splinter, but at least death must have been quick – an accident that medical attention could not have helped. A priest would have been summoned rather than a doctor in this case. So, what was the Church's position on medicine?

2

MEDICINE AND THE CHURCH

In clepynge (calling) Goddes help, he schall conforte ham
and saie that this passioun or sekenesse is salvacioun of the
soule ...

The Cyrurgie, Guy de Chauliac, mid-fourteenth century

In medieval times, illness was believed to be a punishment for
sin and God was reckoned to be the 'Divine Physician' who sent
sickness or healing, depending on His will. For this reason, medical
treatment was more concerned with caring for the sick – especially
their souls – than with curing them. Certain churchmen even
believed that attempting to heal the sick was flouting God's will
and endangering the patient's soul; after all, he must be paying
for some sin he'd committed. The healer's own soul was also
put at risk by trying to deny God's wishes. Fortunately, others
thought that if there was a cure or treatment available, then God
had provided it and not to make use of it was also going against
God's intentions. You can see straight away how medicine could
be both controversial and complicated. Anyone whose views were
different from those of the Roman Catholic Church ran the risk of
being accused of heresy with the dire punishments that entailed.
Therefore, when the Church stated that illnesses were punishments

from God and that those who were ill were so because they were sinners, few dared to argue.

Back in Anglo-Saxon times, medical doctors were most often monks. In the late ninth century, King Alfred's doctor, Bald, was a monk who compiled a leechbook – a treasure trove of medical remedies and advice – that contains, among its numerous recipes, treatments for piles (haemorrhoids) and various aches and pains which tormented the unfortunate monarch. It seems that Bald had practical experience of dealing with the sick and probably learned the basics from a brother monk well versed in the healing arts, doing a kind of apprenticeship in the making of medicines and the carrying out of surgical procedures. From lancing boils and extracting teeth to administering enemas and couching cataracts, the monk would have been quite capable of carrying out these procedures.

In Bald's time there were no universities in the West where he could have trained, although there were medical schools in Alexandria in Egypt and Salerno in Italy where classes were conducted in Greek, not Latin. Bald may have attended one of these. If he did, he would have learned the theories of medicine, based on the idea that 'medicine and philosophy are sisters: that medicine is the philosophy of the body and philosophy the medicine of the soul'.[1] The curriculum would have required him to study the Greek texts of men like Hippocrates and Galen, written centuries before. If this sounds rather involved, the Roman Catholic Church was to make things more difficult still.

The Fourth Lateran Council, convened by Pope Innocent III in 1215, made matters even more complex when it decided that clerics should be forbidden to spill blood. Canon no. 18 was intended to bar churchmen from passing a death sentence if they sat in judgement in a law court, or to prevent them from being 'put in command of mercenaries or crossbowmen or suchlike men of blood'. That seems reasonable enough, but it also stated, 'Nor may a subdeacon, deacon or priest practise the art of surgery, which involves cauterizing and making incisions.'[2] This was important for medicine as it meant that monks, like Bald, and priests, previously the best doctors available, could no longer be surgeons. From now on, surgeons had to be laymen or, occasionally, women. Churchmen might still study to become qualified physicians, learning all the theoretical ideas of medicine from the old textbooks, but they would have no practical training. The possibility of studying human anatomy was almost nonexistent because the Church didn't permit human dissection, so animal anatomy had to provide a stopgap alternative. Pigs were reckoned to be closest in size and structure to man and, being readily available, were most often used for anatomical study. This was the reason why butchers knew more about anatomy, such as it was, than university-trained physicians. However, pigs aren't the same, obviously, and this led to further mysteries, including the inexplicable 'right-side sickness'. We call it appendicitis but pigs don't have an appendix, hence the mystery.

University Education

By the early 1200s, universities were being founded across Europe. Bologna and Paris were among the first; Oxford University was founded in 1167, after King Henry II banned English students from going to Paris, and Cambridge University in 1208 by a group of breakaway scholars from Oxford who fled the town when one of their fellows was murdered there. They also had a few ideas of their own as to how they thought the university should be run. Wherever the universities grew up and however they were set up, throughout Europe they all had one thing in common: they were under Church jurisdiction with the basic intention of training men for the priesthood. This meant that every scholar had to take at least minor holy orders, no woman could ever study at a university and medical training took a back seat, well behind the study of both theology and law. As late as the 1660s, when Isaac Newton wanted to graduate at Cambridge, his unorthodox religious beliefs meant he didn't want to take holy orders of any kind. He had to apply to King Charles II, as head of the Church of England, for special permission to receive his Master's degree without doing so.

The university education of doctors in medieval England consisted of a course lasting from six to nine years at either Oxford or Cambridge, often with some time spent at a foreign university – Salerno and Paris were two of the most renowned and the earliest to specialise in medicine. The course, which would be taught entirely in Latin wherever they studied, consisted of a basic three-year curriculum – the 'trivium' – covering grammar, rhetoric and logic. Alongside the trivium, those who wished to study medicine would cover the basic medical texts of Hippocrates, Aristotle, Galen, Soranus and other noteworthy classical authors, learning great swathes of information by heart. This expanse of knowledge would be used to argue cases with fellow students in discussions supervised by the tutors, relying on their skills in logic and rhetoric to win the debate. Examinations would consist of a series of oral questions, which the student should be able to answer from all that he had learned by rote from the ancient texts.

However, the Church had a particular problem with the writings of both the Greek and the later Roman scholars: these men were pagans, born either before the birth of Christ or before the new religion based on Christ's teaching became accepted across the Roman Empire. How could these sources of knowledge be made acceptable to the Roman Catholic Church and compatible with its own teachings? After due consideration, much prayer and soul-searching, the Church decided that Hippocrates, Galen and the others *would* have been good Christians if only they hadn't suffered the great inconvenience of being born too soon. They were made honorary Christians so scholars could absorb their writings with clear consciences, without endangering their souls in the least. An anonymous late medieval poet wrote this verse, not only proclaiming that Hippocrates, Galen and Socrates – I think he may have meant Soranus, since Socrates didn't practise medicine, as far as I know – 'practised their medicines by God's grace', but begging Christ to accept their souls into the joy of heaven:

> Thus seith Ypocras the goode surgean,
> And Socrates and Galean,
> That wore ffilosophers alle thre
> That tyme the best in any cuntre,
> In this world were noon hure peere
> As far as any man myght here,
> And practisedem medycyns be Godus grace
> To save mannus lyf in dyvers place.
> Cryst that made bothe est and west
> Leve here soules have good reste,
> Evere-more in ioye to be
> In heven with God in trinite.[3]

After successfully completing the trivium, the student would go on to the next stage of his education: the four-year 'quadrivium', which included astronomy, geometry, music and algebra. An understanding of astronomy and geometry was vital because physicians had to draw up astrological charts to assist not only in working out the appropriate treatments for their future patients but also in forecasting the likely outcomes of their ailments. Music, too, was thought to be beneficial to health, such that Anglo-Saxon leechbooks sometimes instructed the doctor to sing to the patient as part of his medical treatment, as in this remedy to treat a fever:

First make an amulet of [communion] wafers, then sing a charm, first in the patient's left ear, then the right and, finally, over the top of the head while hanging the amulet around the patient's neck.[4]

Having settled matters regarding the suitability of the Greek and Roman texts for Christian scholars, Canon no. 22 of the Fourth Lateran Council of 1215 went further in dealing with medical practice, declaring that 'before prescribing for the sick, physicians shall be bound under pain of exclusion from the Church, to exhort their patients to call in a priest, and thus provide for their spiritual welfare'. Obviously, the care of the soul was thought to be far more important than any medical attention.

Bearing in mind the Church's attitude to the sick, the best treatment for any ailment was to prevent it in the first place. The Church taught that the only way to keep healthy was to avoid committing any sins, so God wouldn't punish you by making you suffer pain and illness. If you did become ill, prayer and penance were the first things you tried, hoping God would forgive your sin and you'd quickly recover. But supposing that didn't work?

Pilgrimage as a Medical Treatment

The ultimate penance was to make a pilgrimage to some holy shrine or other. All kinds of people made pilgrimages, some going all the way to Jerusalem. The rich rode horses or even camels; others walked. The lame went on crutches; others carrying their children. In fact, the more difficult the journey, the more credit you earned for your soul in Heaven. If your pilgrimage did not miraculously cure your illness, it was still of great benefit to your soul, which was even more important.

It wasn't necessary to go as far as Jerusalem or even Rome. For Londoners, the favoured destination was the tomb of their fellow Londoner Thomas Becket at Canterbury Cathedral. The journey itself could become more like a holiday, enjoying a good time with the other pilgrims you met along the way, like those in Chaucer's *Canterbury Tales,* which was written in the 1390s.

As souvenirs of the journey, most centres of pilgrimage sold badges, some made of cheap metals for the poor, others gilded for the wealthier pilgrims to buy. Afterwards, the badges were worn not only as mementoes and medals of valour showing what the wearer had achieved but also as religious charms to protect them from all kinds of horrors, from sickness to fire, from robbery to accident.

Walsingham was a popular pilgrimage destination in the south-east of England. The combined villages of Great and Little Walsingham in Norfolk became a major centre of pilgrimage in the eleventh century. In 1061, according to the Walsingham legend, an Anglo-Saxon noblewoman, Richeldis de Faverches, had a vision of the Virgin Mary in which she was instructed to build a replica of the house of the holy family in Nazareth in honour of the Annunciation. When it was built, the holy house was panelled with wood and contained a wooden statue of an enthroned Virgin Mary with the child Jesus seated on her lap. Among its relics was a phial of the Virgin's milk. Walsingham became one of northern Europe's great places of pilgrimage and remained so throughout most of the Middle Ages.

The chapel was founded during the reign of Edward the Confessor, around 1063, the earliest deeds naming Richeldis, the mother of Geoffrey of Faverches, as the founder. In 1169, Geoffrey granted 'to God and St Mary and to Edwy his clerk the chapel of our Lady' which his mother had founded at Walsingham with the intention that Edwy should found a priory. By the time of its destruction in 1538 during the reign of Henry VIII, the shrine had become one of the greatest religious centres in England together with Glastonbury and Canterbury.

Royal patronage helped the shrine to grow in wealth and popularity, receiving visits from Henry III, Edward I, II and III, Henry IV and VI. King Edward IV visited with his queen, Elizabeth Woodville, in 1470 when, with so many daughters, they were desperate for a son and heir. It certainly worked for them so Henry VII and his queen, Elizabeth of York, made the pilgrimage after their eldest son Arthur died. Henry VIII tried it too with both Catherine of Aragon and Anne Boleyn, but no son and heir arrived for them – perhaps reason enough for Henry to close down Walsingham Abbey and the shrine in 1538.

Pilgrimages were a popular 'cure' whatever the ailment, but even if the patient was too sick to make a pilgrimage himself, all was not lost. A friend or relative could make the journey instead and bring back a vial of holy water for the patient. An image showing this is the subject of a stained-glass window in Canterbury Cathedral. If it was too late to think about a personal pilgrimage, folk left money in their wills to pay for others to go on their behalf. In 1471, a London barber-surgeon, Rowland Frankyssh, who seems to have had roots in Yorkshire, left money in his will for his wife Ellen to make a whole series of pilgrimages in his name to include Beverley, York, Guisborough, Bridlington, Walsingham and Canterbury.

The death of the patient in no way detracted from the efficacy of the pilgrimage, which was believed to have posthumous benefits for his soul in purgatory, if not for his physical body. One particular royal case clearly shows this – that of Prince Henry (1155–83), the Young King, eldest son of Henry II. He lay dying of dysentery after despoiling and plundering the monasteries of northern France, and sent his companion, William Marshall, on a crusade-pilgrimage to the Holy Land on his behalf to make restitution for his recent sins, knowing he would be dead himself within a day or two. Henry had vowed to go on crusade personally and had received the official cloak of a crusading knight. Now that couldn't happen. He told his servants to pile penitential ashes on the floor of his chamber and spread the cloak on top of them. Then he lay on the cloak and died there, rather than in his bed. The fact that another man went on the journey to Jerusalem made it no less a pilgrimage in Prince Henry's name for the good of his soul. You have to wonder whether William Marshall earned any spiritual merit for himself, having gone to so much effort on his lord's behalf.

The most popular place of pilgrimage in England was, of course, Canterbury, to visit the shrine of St Thomas Becket in the cathedral. Archbishop Thomas had been murdered before the altar there in December 1170 and was soon being venerated as a saint and martyr capable of miraculous acts of healing. The bloodstained cloak he had been wearing when he was killed was given away to the poor of Canterbury, along with other items of his clothing, in exchange for their prayers for his soul. It seems the monks hadn't yet realised that these weren't just the dead man's unneeded possessions to be given away, but irreplaceable 'holy relics'. However, William, the priest at nearby Bishopsbourne, bought the cloak from its new poor owner and took it home to his little parish church, to exhibit it as a precious relic of Becket's martyrdom. But it wasn't only for show; when the priest wrapped the cloak around a sick child as it lay dying, the infant made a miraculous recovery.[5]

According to Becket's acolyte and biographer William FitzStephen, the archbishop had enacted his first miracle within hours of his murder. A group of citizens had witnessed his slaughter from the gloomy recesses of the nave, not daring to intervene as the four assassins went about their grisly work. Afterwards, the citizens had come forward and dipped their clothes in the martyr's blood. One man took his bloodstained shirt home and told his family, friends and neighbours the news, recounting the gory details, which had them all in tears. His wife suffered from paralysis of some kind, but was a practical woman. She told her husband to soak his shirt in cold water – the best way to remove bloodstains – but 'she thereupon drank [the water] and rose up cured'. FitzStephen claims this was the first miracle wrought by St Thomas – the first of numerous acts of healing catalogued by the monks of Canterbury as future evidence for his canonisation.

Not all pilgrimages were made in order to request a miraculous cure. Sometimes people went on pilgrimage as an act of thanksgiving for a life already saved, an injury healed or a recovery from sickness. One man deemed suitably saintly in the late fifteenth century was King Henry VI. His canonisation in the early sixteenth century never occurred because England split from the Roman Catholic Church before the Pope got around to considering his possible sainthood. Nevertheless, a catalogue of his miracles was kept at Windsor. Miracle number 113 tells the story of nine-month-old Miles Freebridge of London who, as babies do, liked to put anything and everything in his mouth. Unwisely perhaps, Miles had been given a lovely shiny pilgrim badge of St Thomas Becket to play with and immediately tried to swallow it. The badge became stuck in his throat and baby Miles was choking. His father tried to dislodge the badge but only made things worse as his son turned blue and any signs of life faded. Despairing of saving him, the father prayed to the Virgin Mary and 'the most noble King Henry that death might not so overtake his child'. The baby promptly coughed up the badge and breathed again. His grateful parent then made a pilgrimage from London to Windsor to thank the would-be saint, adding this miracle to the catalogue of marvellous cures and leaving that near-lethal badge of St Thomas as an offering.[6] Other miraculous recoveries, similarly recorded and credited to King Henry, included boys who had drowned: six-year-old John Bythewey of Dorchester in Dorset fell into the river while playing with his little brothers, yet revived after three hours with 'his head under water', and the son of Richard Woodward of Kennington in Kent 'escaped free from the same pains of death'.

The medical profession agreed on the healing possibilities of a pilgrimage. The London surgeon Richard Esty, who became Upper Warden of the Surgeons' Guild in 1459 and again in 1463–64, included a section on the subject in his medical handbook written in 1454.[7] This incredible manuscript, now in the Wellcome Library for the History and Understanding of Medicine in London, describes in detail the pilgrim route from London, via Calais,

Pavia in Italy, Venice, Corfu, Rhodes and Jaffa, all the way to Jerusalem, with helpful information on overnight stops, money exchange rates and pitfalls for the traveller to avoid. Esty listed the 'indulgence value' (that is, time off earned in lieu for the soul when it entered purgatory after death) of the numerous places the pilgrim could visit in the Holy Land, from the pool where 'our lady wascht the clothis of our lord Jehsu Criste in hys childhod' to the 'kave where Jesu Criste was borne, layd be twyx a nox & a nasse' in Bethlehem to the Garden of Gethsemane.

So, how did medieval medicine explain these miraculous cures brought about by prayer, pilgrimage or contact of some kind with holy relics? The answer is that it didn't. It did not need to; physicians and surgeons accepted that miracles happened sometimes and prayers were as valid a treatment as a change of diet or a herbal remedy and, of course, had Church backing. In some cases, as with plague, a miracle cure was the patient's best hope, or, knowing the dangers lurking in certain treatments, prayer was the safest option. In a far more cynical age, we expect medical science to be able to explain any unexpected recovery, but even today this isn't always possible. Some 'miracles' may well have been brought about by the placebo effect, recognised as a genuine phenomenon by modern science – give the patient some treatment, real or not, tell him he will feel better because of it and he does.

A twentieth-century example of the placebo effect was recorded by anaesthetist Henry Beecher during the Second World War. A badly wounded soldier was about to undergo major surgery, but the supply of morphine had run out. When the soldier was given an injection of simple saline solution he relaxed, ready for surgery, and seemed to feel very little pain during the operation. Neither did he go into shock, as would have been expected without any anaesthetic.[8] In the fifteenth century, this would have been accounted a miracle requiring no further explanation, but nowadays we want science to tell us how this could be so.

The Automaton at Boxley Abbey

For pilgrims on their way to Canterbury, there was the opportunity to take a brief detour to visit Boxley Abbey near Maidstone in Kent. St Mary's Abbey there was famous for its miraculous Holy Rood, an image of Christ upon the cross which was said to move its eyes, lips and limbs. Prayers and offerings made before this image were believed to effect miraculous cures. Before Henry VIII dissolved the monasteries – Boxley's 'abbey of the Holy Cross of Grace' was dissolved in February 1538 – the Rood was venerated by the great and good. Henry VII sent four shillings to the abbey in 1492. Then, in 1502, when she was too ill to travel in person, Henry's queen, Elizabeth of York, sent one of her chaplains, Richard Milner, there to make a donation of 1s 8d in the hope that a cure would be granted to her.

Shortly before the Dissolution of the Monasteries, Archbishop Warham of Canterbury wrote to Cardinal Wolsey in connection with claims being made against Boxley Abbey, as Henry VIII was looking for reasons to close it down. Warham told the cardinal that '[the abbey] was much sought after by visitors to the Rood from all parts of the realm, and so he would be sorry to put it under an interdict'. He called it 'so holy a place where so many miracles be showed'.[9] But Warham's reluctance was ignored and Boxley was stripped of all its assets, including the miraculous Rood. The more fanatical supporters of the new Protestant religion found, to their delight, that inside the Rood were bits of string and sticks and pulleys which were parts of an ancient mechanism for moving the figure of Christ. The monks claimed to know nothing of it and it was in a state of disrepair, looking unused for decades, but Thomas Cromwell, mastermind of the dissolution, took full advantage of the discovery to 'prove' that the Roman Catholic Church had defrauded the people of their donations, perpetrating the lie of the marvellous image:

Which image was made of paper and clouts from the legs

upward; each leg and arms were of timber. And so the people had been deluded and caused to do great idolatry by the said image, of long continuance, to the derogation of God.[10]

The image was taken into the nearby town of Maidstone, where it was market day, and the locals were shown how they had all been fooled. The Rood then went to London, and in St Paul's Cathedral the Protestant Bishop of Rochester explained all the trickery to the people, as an eyewitness explained:

By means of some person pulling a cord, most artfully contrived and ingeniously inserted at the back, the image rolled about its eyes just like a living creature; and on the pulling of other cords it gave a nod of assent or dissent according to the occasion. It never restored health to any sick person, notwithstanding great numbers afflicted with divers diseases were carried to it, and laid prostrate before it, unless some one disguised himself of set purpose, and pretended to be sick; in which case it would give a nod, as though promising the restoration of health, that it might by this means confirm its imposture. Then, again, by some contrivance unknown to me, it opened and shut its mouth; and to make an end of my story at once, after all its tricks had been exposed to the people, it was broken into small pieces.[11]

The monks' accusers weren't content to describe the Rood as it was, but invented new details saying it was capable of smiling, frowning, weeping and grimacing. Although such things were impossible, they were necessary to make it more outlandish still, seeing that the pilgrims to Boxley were not lowly country bumpkins, easily fooled, but lords and ladies, kings and queens, bishops and archbishops. And it had to be made plausible how all these intelligent people could have been taken in by this fraudulent object. Popish trickery was the Protestants' explanation. Yet the monks of Boxley had always told the intriguing story that the Rood had been brought to the abbey by a carpenter's runaway horse. They admitted it was the work of a humble artisan, from whom they bought the image which had arrived so unexpectedly on their doorstep, seeing God had meant them to have it. That the cleverly constructed machine attracted pilgrims who put money in the abbey coffers was a fortunate bonus – a financial miracle, perhaps, but not a healing one. The monks protested that they had never claimed it could cure sickness or disability. Despite this, as Archbishop Warham had told Wolsey, Boxley was 'where so many miracles be showed'.

So, were people taken in by this kind of mechanical device? Probably not. The world's first 'vending machine' had been constructed for religious purposes in around AD 50 by the Greek engineer Hero of Alexandria. In return for a coin, the machine dispensed holy water to visitors to the Egyptian city. Automatons were known in medieval times and some of the scenery and props used in the popular mystery plays involved ropes and pulleys to operate such things as the serpent in the Garden of Eden, hell's mouth and a dove to fly down at Pentecost.[12] Without understanding the intricate engineering such things were baffling, but not miraculous; something to enthrall the spectators. Alderman Gosiman of Hull left instructions in his will of 1502 that £40 of his money was to be used in the construction, at the high altar of his parish church, of 'some machinery by which angels should ascend to the roof of the church and descend again, from the elevation of the Sacred Host to the end of the Pater Noster'.[13]

Miracle Cures by Patron Saints

Another option, open not only to the patient but to those treating him, was to make prayers to an appropriate patron saint. In medieval times, everyone had a patron saint. They might choose one whose special day was closest to the date on which they were born, or with whom they shared a name or even a trade. Physicians had the choice of either St Luke, one of Christ's apostles, or St Cosmas. Conveniently, Cosmas's twin brother, St Damian, was the patron saint of surgeons, so between them they had medical practice sewn up. This was just as well because their most famous miracle was performed when the saintly physician and his surgeon brother performed the first ever limb transplant, assisted by angels. In an exquisite illuminated miniature the operation is shown in progress, but unfortunately for the pale-skinned patient his gangrenous leg is being replaced by that of an African – not a good colour match, but a miraculous hint at the future of medicine.

Cosmas and Damian were early Christians whose feast day is celebrated on 27 September. They were born in Arabia[14] and practised their healing arts in the seaport of Aegea, in Asia Minor. They accepted no payment for their services and attracted the attention of the Roman authorities at a time when Christianity was outlawed. The brothers were arrested and tortured but, miraculously, suffered no injury from 'water, fire, air, nor on the cross'. Finally, they were beheaded with a sword on 27 September AD 287. Their remains were buried in the city of Cyrus in Syria. More than two centuries later, the Emperor Justinian (527–65) was cured of a serious illness after praying to the saints and, in gratitude for their aid, rebuilt and adorned their church at Constantinople, which became a celebrated place of pilgrimage. In Rome, there is another church dedicated to Cosmas and Damian which has the most beautiful mosaics and is still a place of pilgrimage today.

If a patient preferred a saint a little closer to home, he might have prayed to Bishop Hugh of Lincoln, the patron saint of sick people, particularly of sick children, and the second most popular English saint after St Thomas Becket. He was also the patron saint of shoemakers and of swans, a bird he kept as a pet and which became his symbol. According to Adam of Eynsham, a monk who wrote a biography of the bishop, Hugh was so pious that he had miraculously healed lepers with a kiss and raised children from the dead. After his death, it was said that every sick person who attended Bishop Hugh's funeral in the year 1200, in Lincoln Cathedral, was healed by the time they got home afterwards. Only Hugh's pet swan pined away and died soon after.

The Knights Hospitaller

The Knights Hospitaller seem to have begun as a group of Benedictine monks working at a hospital in Jerusalem which was dedicated to St John the Baptist. The hospital had been founded around 1023 to provide care for poor, sick or injured pilgrims to the Holy Land. After the forces of Islam had seized Jerusalem, the Christians were determined to take back their most revered sites, so in 1099 they organised the First Crusade to reclaim the Holy Land. The First Crusade was successful in retaking Jerusalem, but the area was never again entirely at peace. At first the Knights Hospitaller cared for pilgrims in Jerusalem, but they became the military Order of St John with a papal charter, issued in 1113, that decreed the knights should protect and defend the Holy Land itself, as well as giving safe escort to pilgrims passing through.[15]

The order distinguished itself in battle against the Muslims, its soldiers wearing a black surcoat with a white cross – a badge still worn today by the St John's Ambulance Brigade, the non-military first-aiders who are the order's modern descendants. In the late twelfth century, the order had gained recognition in England and set up priories, called commanderies, on land donated to the order by local nobles. However, the power of Islam eventually took back Jerusalem in 1187 and the rest of the Holy Land fell to the Muslims, bit by bit. Seeking refuge on the island of Cyprus, the Knights Hospitaller became entangled in the local politics and moved on to the island of Rhodes. It took two years of besieging the island, but in August 1309 the inhabitants finally surrendered and Rhodes became the Hospitallers' new home.

Although they had become a military force to be reckoned with, the Knights Hospitaller of St John hadn't forgotten their original intentions of tending the sick and injured. On the beaches of their island home they found strange pinkish pebbles, some of which were clearly marked with a black cross. Obviously, so they thought, these 'stones of Rhodes' had been sent especially by God, bearing the sign of the cross, for the Hospitallers' use. Stories evolved that told of the pebbles' powers of protection and healing, and visiting pilgrims, on their way to face dangers ranging from Barbary pirates and Muslim marauders to scorpions and heat stroke, were eager to buy the holy pebbles as talismans. Pebbles found their way back to England in pilgrims' purses and became eagerly sought after to ward off plague and cure any number of lesser ailments. This kind of medical 'treatment' had the full support of the Church and the Hospitallers made money from exporting their intriguing little stones for sale by apothecaries and itinerant peddlers across Europe.

The stones still exist, although they are now mined as 'rhodonite' in many places, from Sweden to the USA, so they are not unique to Rhodes, nor were they a gift from God specifically for the Hospitallers to make money. Although their protective and curative powers have yet to be proved, they do sometimes have a cross shape that goes right the way through the stone and they do make attractive pendants when polished. Technically the stones are of manganese silicate,[16] which rather destroys their element of mystery.

It is clear that the Church was powerful in determining just how medicine was practised, but did religion influence what a doctor learned during his education and training? And what exactly did he have to study?

3

ADAM KNEW EVERYTHING!

And the Lord God ... brought them to Adam to see what he would call them; for whatsoever Adam called any living creature the same is its name.

King James Bible, Genesis 2:19

In the beginning, God created Adam, and Adam knew everything.

That was what medieval scholars believed, convinced that Adam had known everything there was to know. In the Bible, in Genesis 2:19–20, God brought all the birds and beasts before Adam for him to name them. Presumably, Adam was also given the job of naming every plant, rock and geographical feature on earth as well. In medieval terms, 'naming' someone or something meant knowing everything about that person or object – the naming of a baby at its baptism made it known entirely to and recognised by God.

The problems began when Eve had her encounter with the Devil in the Garden of Eden and the perfect couple decided to sample the fruit of the tree of knowledge, despite God's command that they must not – they might eat any other fruit except that one. Not so perfect any longer, Adam and Eve produced offspring, every generation a little less perfect than their parents. As a result, they not only began to suffer from various ailments and eventually died, but also their memories were no longer infallible either. This meant each subsequent generation in the 5,000 years or so since the Creation[1] had forgotten a little more of Adam's encyclopaedic knowledge and passed on a little less to their children.

Eventually, by medieval times, scholars believed mankind had become deplorably ignorant. Far from assuming, as we do today, that knowledge increases as we discover more and more about life, the universe and medicine in particular, they viewed the matter in reverse: knowledge was diminishing. The answer was to go back to the earliest known written sources to recover what had been lost.[2]

By the twelfth century, texts from ancient Greece were becoming known in western Europe, the writings of men like Hippocrates, Socrates, Pythagoras and Aristotle from the time before the birth of Christ. Obviously, to the medieval way of thinking these men must have known so much more, having had far fewer preceding generations to forget Adam's vital information. Therefore, to study medicine, or any other subject, properly involved a thorough and comprehensive knowledge of the ancient sources. As we saw in chapter 2, the universities were at the centre of this pool of knowledge, so what did the ancient sources teach about the subject of medicine?

Claudius Galen's Theory of the Four Humours

One of the basic ideas in medieval medicine was the theory of the 'Four Humours', which the Greco-Roman writer Claudius Galen (c. AD 129–216), also known as the 'Prince of Physicians', covered in great detail in his medical books. Galen was born in the city of Pergamon to Greek parents. His father was an architect but in a dream he was 'told' to see that his son trained to become a physician. Sixteen-year-old Galen was particularly interested in anatomy and spent some time at the medical school in Alexandria, where a human skeleton was available for study.[2] Human dissection was generally forbidden in both classical and later Christian cultures, as mentioned in chapter 2. Back home in

Pergamon, now aged thirty, Galen was appointed as physician and surgeon to the gladiators. Attending wounded gladiators must have given him more opportunities than most to see how the human body was constructed, their severe injuries acting like windows into their insides. His surgical skills became famous, especially since he succeeded in saving the lives of many more valuable gladiators than his predecessors had done.[3] Ambitious for more, Galen moved to Rome, where Marcus Aurelius Antoninus had recently become emperor and Galen was swiftly appointed as the imperial physician.

Galen had been in Rome for just a few years when 'a plague' broke out in AD 165. This was most probably an epidemic of smallpox, variously known as the Antonine Plague (after the emperor's full name) or as the 'Plague of Galen' because the physician wrote about the terrible effects of the epidemic on the Roman Empire and its people. Perhaps as many as five million people died of the smallpox during the fifteen years that the plague lasted, the emperor himself perhaps one of the last to succumb to the disease in AD 180, despite Galen's best efforts no doubt.

In spite of his duties as the imperial physician, Galen managed to find the time to write a vast amount about medicine on his own account, as well as expanding on the writings attributed to Hippocrates, the 'Father of Medicine', and to Aristotle. Following their lead, Galen described how the human body, like everything else in their world, was made up of the four elements: earth, air, fire and water. In mankind, these elements combined to form the four humours: blood, phlegm, yellow and black bile. An anonymous poem of the fifteenth century shows us that these ideas were still current over a thousand years later:

God made all mankind that lives on earth
Of four elements, as we in books read:
Of fire and of air, of water and of erthe,
That [en]genders in us humours, as Aristotle us learns [*sic*].[4]

According to Galen's theories, everyone had a natural excess of one or other, making them sanguine, phlegmatic, choleric or melancholy. In a healthy individual these humours were pretty well in balance, but if they became too unbalanced, as a result of lifestyle or environmental influences, then the patient fell ill. The humours gave off vapours which rose up into the brain, affecting the temperament, so a good physician could work out the problem by looking at the person's complexion: a sanguine individual was happy, cheerful, amorous and generous. Obviously, this wouldn't seem to be too much of a problem and was usually reckoned the most acceptable imbalance, unless the patient became hysterically happy or sex-mad. A choleric individual tended to be easily angered, violent and argumentative, melancholy people were gluttonous, lazy and miserable, while phlegmatic people were dull, pale, cowardly and not particularly bothered about anything. Sickness was believed to be the result if the humours strayed too far out of balance.

Below is a table showing the 'qualities' associated with the four elements, the humours and human temperaments derived from them:

Element	Qualities	Humour	Temperament
Fire	Hot & dry	Choler or yellow bile	Choleric
Air	Hot & wet	Blood	Sanguine
Water	Cold & wet	Phlegm	Phlegmatic
Earth	Cold & dry	Black bile	Melancholic

If a patient's humours were just a little off balance, the physician would prescribe a suitable diet to adjust them. Too phlegmatic – cold and moist – he would prescribe something hot and dry like spicy beef. Too choleric – hot and dry – a fish diet would be advised. Humours were also affected by the seasons. A good example of how this theory was seen to work in practice was the medieval understanding of the common cold. Then as now, the winter months saw an increase in the incidence of upper respiratory tract infections – colds. Using the theories of the time, this condition, characterised by a runny nose, a cough and generally feeling low, was thought to be caused by an excess of phlegm within the body. This in turn was explained by the colder winter weather, with the icy wind and rain exerting their adverse environmental influences on the body, leading to an imbalance of the four vital elements: too much cold air and water means too much phlegm. Conversely, the heat and dryness of summer caused a rise in choleric hot tempers and fevers.

An unsuitable diet, too much wine or too much sex, too much or too little sleep or exercise, or exposure to those fearful 'miasmas' that penetrated the body, causing disease to develop, could disrupt a good, healthy balance of the humours. If changing the patient's diet or lifestyle didn't work to restore his health, then more drastic steps were needed; bloodletting and possibly medication would follow. The same rules were used to work out what would be the right treatment for the patient. If he needed them, medications with an equal and opposite effect would be prescribed to restore the balance of his humours.

King Henry VI of England suffered a long period of mental illness in 1453–55, when he fell into a stupor, unable to speak or recognise anyone. His condition may have been genetic in origin: his grandfather Charles VI of France went quite mad in his later years. Believing he was made of glass, Charles refused to allow anyone to touch him, fearing he would shatter if they did – how terrifying that must have been for the unfortunate king. Meanwhile, in England, Henry's physicians and surgeons used a whole range of treatments. In order to restore his balance of humours he was given warm baths and purges (enemas and/or emetics) and was bled. His diet was carefully regulated to reduce the cold, wet phlegmatic humours that rose into his brain and caused the problem. He was fed hot food, like spiced chicken broth, but it was eighteen months before he regained his faculties. His recovery wasn't permanent either; the king continued to suffer from periodic mental illness until his death in 1471.

Some Surprisingly Modern Ideas

Occasionally, alongside ideas that seem so wide of the mark, there was sometimes a surprisingly modern one that was right on target. In the first century AD, the Roman philosopher and writer Aulus Celsus (25 BC – AD 50), when writing about rabies, used the word 'virus' in connection with dog bites. In Latin *virus* means 'something slimy and poisonous'. Celsus suggested that if anyone was bitten by a rabid dog, 'the virus must be drawn out with a cupping glass'.[5] As it happens, Celsus had the right word for the infection, even though it was not until the 1930s that any 'virus' – a tiny micro-organism that can only reproduce inside another living cell – was actually 'seen' using an electron microscope. He was correct in using the term in that rabies *is* caused by a virus rather than a bacterium.   *isn't this rather serendipitous reasoning?*

Even the concept of clinical trials was not entirely unknown, although they were hardly conducted according to the scientific principles demanded today. The Book of Daniel in the Old Testament tells how Daniel conducted a ten-day dietary experiment, using a control group to compare the results. He wanted to prove that the vegetarian diet he and his friends ate would keep them as fit and healthy looking, if not in better shape, than if they ate the sumptuous royal food that King Nebuchadnezzar wanted to feed to his noble Jewish captives. Daniel was warned that the king would be angry if his prisoners looked gaunt and skinny, but the vegetarian group won the contest in healthy looks: 'And at the end of ten days their countenances appeared fairer and fatter in flesh than all the children which did eat the portion of the king's meat.'[6]

The outcome was assessed subjectively rather than mathematically, as in a modern clinical trial, but the idea of comparative results was there. With this biblical precedent, did that mean the Church could approve of experimental research? It seems unlikely. We know of hardly any similar experiments carried out in medieval times and some that were conducted most certainly wouldn't have had support from the Church.

The Holy Roman Emperor Frederick II (r. 1220–50) had a keen interest in science and is alleged to have carried out some horrifying human experiments which were recorded by a monk. Despite the fact that the Pope had been Frederick's guardian when he was orphaned as a boy and conducted his coronation as emperor, Frederick admitted to being a religious sceptic. Not surprisingly, the monkish chronicler Salimbene, from whom we learn of the emperor's scientific interests, despised the man so this may have coloured his reporting. One experiment involved sealing a prisoner inside a cask until he died, a close watch being kept to see if the soul could be observed escaping though a hole in the barrel.

Frederick also wondered about the effects of sleep and exercise on a man's digestion. He had two prisoners served identical dinners, then sent one to bed and the other out hunting. A few hours later, Frederick had both men killed and disembowelled. Their stomach contents were then examined to see how the digestive process had progressed. The Church could not have sanctioned such slaughter in the name of science. Incidentally, as a matter of academic interest, the imperial physicians determined that the man who went hunting hadn't digested his meal to the extent of the prisoner who spent his final hours of life asleep. The fact that he was able to sleep at all suggests the prisoners had no idea how the trial would be concluded.

Another of the emperor's interests was the origin of language. To study this, Frederick had infants imprisoned from birth and kept them without any kind of verbal contact to see if they would develop a language naturally and what language that might be, hoping to discover which language God had given to Adam and Eve. The unfortunate babies were raised with the minimum of human interaction. Salimbene wrote that the emperor ordered the 'foster-mothers and nurses to suckle and bathe and wash the children, but in no ways to prattle or speak with them' to see whether they would speak Hebrew, Greek, Latin or Arabic, or else the language of the parents to whom they had been born. The monk continues: 'But he laboured in vain, for the children could not live without clappings of the hands and gestures and gladness of countenance and blandishments.'[7]

Frederick's scientific 'research' included a great interest in astrology and astronomy and he corresponded with the leading scholars of the day, asking questions on science, mathematics and physics. He also wrote a book himself on falconry. Titled *The Art of Hunting with Birds* (in Latin: *De Arte Venandi cum Avibus*), this was an academic text described by the historian Charles H. Haskins as

a scientific book, approaching the subject from Aristotle but based closely on observation and experiment throughout, *Divisivus et Inquisitivus*, in the words of the preface; it is at the same time a scholastic book, minute and almost mechanical in its divisions and subdivisions. It is also a rigidly practical book, written by a falconer for falconers and condensing a long experience into systematic form for the use of others.[8]

So Frederick was no ignoramus and, in 1224, he founded the University of Naples, the world's oldest university and now called the Università Frederico II in honour of its founder.

Who Was in Charge of Medical Matters?

Medieval medicine was in the hands of physicians, surgeons, barber-surgeons and apothecaries, but why and how were these medical practitioners different from each other? To put it simply, the physicians were educated at university, learning all the theoretical stuff, and were concerned to treat the patient's internal disposition. Surgeons and barber-surgeons – grouped together because giving a man's beard a close shave required the same expertise and equipment as bleeding him or lancing a boil – learned by doing an apprenticeship, acquiring practical knowledge by assisting someone already skilled in the arts of external treatments. This internal/external rule of thumb for dividing physicians and surgeons wasn't entirely logical: drawing up horoscopes was in the physician's remit, while extracting teeth and administering enemas required the surgeon's abilities. Apothecaries also served apprenticeships, learning the secrets of making up medicines.

In theory, if you felt unwell you would call on the services of a physician. He would assess your condition by various means, which are described in more detail in chapter 4. If he decided you needed medical intervention, such as bleeding or amputation, he would give you a prescription to take to a surgeon. If you required a medicine or an ointment, again he would write a prescription, but this time for the services of an apothecary. If you had a wound in your hand that required stitches, or thought you might have fractured your arm, you could go straight to a surgeon who would suture or splint the injury as required but, as with the physician, if he thought you needed a healing ointment or something to ease the pain, he too would write a prescription for the apothecary to make up. If your problem was quite minor – a headache, sore throat or chilblains, perhaps – you could save money by going directly to the apothecary without a prescription. Like a modern pharmacist, the apothecary could sell over-the-counter remedies directly to you, the difference being that no drug was considered too dangerous to sell without a physician's direction. Everything from hemlock to cat's dung was available as a medication without prescription. On the other hand, it wasn't uncommon for both physicians and surgeons to make up their own medicines.

As you can see, there was plenty of scope in this haphazard arrangement for those practising medicine in one way or another to impinge on each others' territories, especially with patients being free to pick and choose how and by whom they would be treated. Following the rules to the letter could also be very expensive, paying separate fees to each practitioner, so patients would frequently cut across the system to save money. In London, matters were further complicated by the guilds. The apothecaries came under the jurisdiction of the Grocers' Company because many of their products were imported by merchants in bulk, or *en gross*, such as sugar, cinnamon and liquorice – items which counted as luxury foodstuffs as well as medications. But the physicians had to ensure that any medicines which the apothecaries made up according to their prescriptions were of good quality, so they wanted to appoint their own inspectors, disregarding those of the Grocers' Company. The Company of Barber-Surgeons was independent too and had its inspectors to guarantee standards of surgical practice in the city, but again the physicians wanted assurance regarding procedures carried out, following their prescriptions. The surgeons also needed to know that the products they purchased from the apothecaries were of a high standard; no point in cleansing and stitching a patient's wound if the apothecary's ointment to smear on it was going to cause it to fester rather than heal. No wonder things were so confusing.

In England, there was just one serious attempt at cooperation between the physicians and surgeons with the foundation of a joint College of Physicians and Surgeons in the City of London in 1423. Sadly, the college was undermined by the powerful Company of Barber-Surgeons, which wanted the surgeons back under its own auspices,[9] and the Grocers' Company, which resented the college's efforts to police the craft of the apothecaries who belonged to their guild. However, for the year or so of its existence, the College of Physicians and Surgeons functioned effectively, having sworn in two official surveyors of surgery, one of whom was the royal surgeon, Thomas Morstede, and two surveyors of physic, along with Gilbert Kymer, personal physician to the king's uncle, Humphrey, Duke of Gloucester, as Rector of Medicines of London.[10] In *The Ordenaunce and Articles of Phisicions withinne the Cite of London and Surgeons of the same cite,* the rules were set out in detail: how the college was to oversee all aspects of practice, who was eligible to work within the city, the paying of fines for malpractice or inappropriate behaviour and the charges made for treatment: 'That none of ye Phisicians ne Cirurgeans take ouer moche mone, or vnresonabely, of eny seke [man].'[11]

The foundation of this short-lived college – it was ended in 1425 – not only showed a willingness to cooperate between physicians and surgeons, but was a public declaration of their desire to be seen as true professionals. It seems that the college was set up as the result of discussions between the royal physician Gilbert Kymer and the royal surgeon Thomas Morstede. Surprisingly, its comprehensive ordinances and petition to the mayor and aldermen of the city were the first guild documents ever to be written in English,[12] perhaps to make it easier for the public to understand the intention of the college to be open and 'honeste' with regard to treating the sick.

The differences between physic and surgery were still recognised in that the ordinance refers to the *Faculte* of Phisyk but the *Crafte* of Cirurgye, denoting the difference in methods of training – university education as against apprenticeship – but this wasn't seen as an insuperable barrier to cooperation between the two; not during the fifteenth century, at least. (The two groups would become bitter rivals in the sixteenth century, after the foundation of the elitist College of Physicians in 1518 which snubbed the surgeons in particular – see chapter 11.) Once beyond the initial training, the college regulations were the same for practitioners in each field: two surveyors of physic, two surveyors of surgery and two apothecaries, all reporting back to the rector, were to police their appropriate practitioners. The apothecary inspectors were to declare 'eny false Medicyns ... in ye Shoppe of eny Apotechary [*sic*] ... withinne ye boundes of London'. Any examples of malpractice were to be taken before the Lord Mayor of London, with the appropriate fines imposed.

There were certainly times when the apothecaries needed to be policed. In 1475, John Davy of London was found to be selling expensive sandalwood which he had concocted himself. Sandalwood was an exotic perfumed wood, usually sold as a reddish powder which was used as a scent and also as a food colouring and flavouring. Davy was fined, put in the pillory for a while and imprisoned. Quite what he had used to make the fake sandalwood powder isn't specified, but something like brick dust would have looked the part. Another apothecary, William of Lothbury, imported a barrel of 'putrid wolves' which he claimed to be a treatment for the 'wolf disease'. Physicians were called to investigate Lothbury's claims, but despite searching their medical textbooks, they couldn't find any disease for which rotting wolf carcasses might be a treatment, so the apothecary had to pay a hefty fine for stocking and trying to sell his revolting 'medication'.[13]

When the Fellowship of Surgeons was set up in 1435, a decade after the failure of the conjoined college, again Thomas Morstede was one of the prime instigators of the ordinances, along with William Bradwardine and fifteen other surgeons of note.[14] Again, the fellowship was intended to police its members – surgeons only in this case – setting out in detail the consequences of malpractice in 'Of peynes of mysgouernaunce' in its regulations. The regulations also covered apprenticeship and as an example of cooperation of a more personal kind, John Dagvile's will of 1477 required his executors to see to the needs of his apprentice William

Hert within eight days of his death. He also specified that at the end of his term of apprenticeship, the executors should present Hert to the Chamberlain of London, as required, in order 'to be sworn and admitted into the fredoms, libertees and fraunchises of the Citee of London'.[15]

Physicians

As we have seen, studying at a university meant the scholar had to take holy orders. John Argentine was born in 1442 and went to school at Eton. He then studied theology at King's College, Cambridge, but having gained his MA it seems he went to Italy, possibly to Ferrara or Padua, to study medicine from 1473 to 1476.[16] This was a common option for continuing an Englishman's education in medicine and was taken by Thomas Linacre among others, one of the co-founders of the College of Physicians in London in 1518,[17] who studied medicine at the University of Padua during the 1490s. When he returned to England, John Argentine took up a number of wealthy benefices as a priest and was also appointed as physician to Edward, Prince of Wales, the elder son of Edward IV, and later served Prince Arthur, the elder son of Henry VII, in the same capacity. Argentine became provost of King's College, Cambridge, in 1501. He wrote a commonplace book containing medical recipes that is now in Oxford, at the Ashmolean Museum, while much of his library went to Gloucester Cathedral. Because he had taken holy orders, Argentine never married; this was the case for many physicians, but not all.

For example, another medical man of note, William Hattecliffe, a physician and a diplomat, did marry. Hattecliffe began his training at Peterhouse, Cambridge, in June 1437 and took holy orders at King's College in 1442. In January 1446, he went to study medicine at Padua, where he received his MD on 5 March 1447. By November 1452, Hattecliffe was one of King Henry VI's physicians, being granted £40 per annum, and on 15 March 1454 he was among the doctors commissioned to attend the Lancastrian king during his months of mental illness, when the king 'barely ever roused from a state of stupor'.

By March 1457, Hattecliffe was also physician to Queen Margaret of Anjou, but by the beginning of 1461 he had apparently joined the Yorkists, this being the time of the Wars of the Roses, contested by the rival royal houses of Lancaster and York. After the Lancastrian victory at the Second Battle of St Albans, also in 1461, Hattecliffe tried to flee to Ireland, but his ship was captured by the French. The new Yorkist king, Edward IV, contributed to Hattecliffe's ransom and in January 1462 he was granted his fee as the king's physician, backdated to the first day of the new reign. Hattecliffe was first employed on diplomatic missions in September 1464, when he was sent to negotiate a treaty with François, Duke of Brittany. By January 1466 he had become one of the king's secretaries – an unusual change of career that may owe something to his acquaintance with Henry Sharpe, the king's protonotary (a lawyer).[18]

Over the next decade Hattecliffe was frequently busy on diplomatic missions without giving up his medical interests. He seems to have specialised in negotiations with Burgundy and the German Hanse merchants, but also had dealings with Denmark and Scotland. During the brief readeption of Henry VI in 1470–71, Hattecliffe was imprisoned and in danger of being executed, but on Edward's return to the throne the physician was restored to his former position, made master of requests and a royal councillor. He had links with the queen's circle – the Woodville family – and in 1473 was acting with the queen on behalf of her kinswoman Anne Haute. He also attended Edward IV to France in 1475, along with other physicians and surgeons. His last diplomatic mission was in 1476, after which the king's French secretary, Oliver King, took over his duties.

Despite having taken minor holy orders, we know William

Hattecliffe was married because the records show that he and his wife Elizabeth retired from London to a house in Westminster in 1478, although this is the only reference to her. Her husband died at their Westminster home in 1480 and was buried in the Lady Chapel of Westminster Abbey. He died a rich man, owning property on the south bank of the Thames and in Greenwich, Deptford and Rotherhithe.[19]

John Crophill of Wix in Essex was an example of a well-educated, part-time, rural practitioner who supplemented his medical work by serving as the bailiff of Wix Priory from 1455 until at least 1477. He compiled a medical book,[20] part of which he wrote himself, the rest being dictated to a scribe. The book contained information taken from both classical and English sources, showing evidence of his wide and varied education, although we don't know how he was trained or where he studied. As his biographer, James Mustain, says, Crophill's standard of medical practice 'perhaps differed little from that provided by the university-trained physician',[21] although his patients were mostly farm labourers and minor craftsmen, some of whom couldn't afford to pay for his services. Crophill must have had a keen sense of vocation, continuing to treat his poorer patients without reward.

Regardless of the way the medical profession was supposed to be organised, with physicians, surgeons and apothecaries being quite separate, each with their own job specifications, on paper at least, the divisions could be blurred. Some physicians made their own medications, without troubling an apothecary for his services, but we know that sometimes the relationship between a physician and his favoured apothecary could be a close one. The Oxford-trained London physician William Goldwyn made his will in June 1482, leaving money for the repair of his parish church of St Stephen in Walbrook.[22] Like many other physicians, having taken holy orders, William wasn't married, so he nominated his mother, Alice Goldwyn, and John Berell, 'apotecary of London', as his executors, so John must have been a trustworthy friend. Goldwyn leaves the apothecary ten marks for his trouble, bequeathing John's wife a 'piece of Paris silver' with a lid and twenty shillings to John's servant, Rose (although we don't know if 'Rose' was a woman's first name or a man's surname).

Surgeons

To become a surgeon Thomas Morstede was apprenticed to the London surgeon Thomas Dayron, and is first recorded as a 'leech' in a deed of 1401.[23] Dayron bequeathed his one-time apprentice two books on surgery and physic when he died in 1407. By 1410, we know that Morstede was in service to Henry IV, but he may have been in royal service as early as 1403, perhaps as an assistant to King's Surgeon John Bradmore (see chapter 9). Together with the surgeon William Bradwardine, Morstede was contracted to serve Henry V on the Agincourt campaign, each of them to bring a team of surgeons and makers of surgical instruments. In 1416, King Henry ordered Morstede and Bradwardine to 'provide without delay for the making of certain instruments necessary and fitting for your mystery', suggesting the surgeons themselves were trained in the crafting of fine tools for surgical use: scalpels, known as fleams, needles for suturing, etc. From his will, written in April 1450, we know Morstede was married at least twice: his first wife, Juliane, predeceased him, and his second wife, Elizabeth, was his widow. Not having to take holy orders, surgeons were free to marry.

An exception to many rules, William Hobbys had an education and training that was hardly typical among the medical fraternity of the fifteenth century. He studied at both Oxford and Cambridge universities, as well as training, by means of an apprenticeship, as a surgeon, possibly under the tutelage of his father, John Hobbys. The Oxford records show that William received his Bachelor of Medicine degree in January 1459, having studied for three years, although he had been 'practising' for twelve years. This was a very rapid graduation as Oxford candidates for a Doctorate of Medicine were expected to gain their Bachelor's degree by attending lectures for eight years – reduced to six for individuals with other relevant qualifications[24] – so Hobbys's knowledge of surgery must have made him an exceptional student.

Having read the usual classical medical texts of Hippocrates and Galen, William would have also studied more contemporary texts, like the *Antidotarium* by Nicholas of Salerno and *De Febribus* (*On Fevers*) by Isaac Judaeus. Anatomy, if it was studied at all by a would-be physician, tended to be in diagrammatic form rather than hands-on dissection. The subject was thought to be far more relevant to surgery, although even in this case it was often studied by means of illustrated books and rarely, if ever, from the examination of a human body. Although keen students might have the opportunity to study animal carcasses, this wasn't an indispensable part of a surgeon's apprenticeship. The art of phlebotomy, either by means of leeches, venous section or 'cupping' (a method of bleeding thought to be less drastic and, therefore, used on children, pregnant women and the elderly), and the application of 'clysters' (or enemas) were considered the more important areas of expertise that a surgeon should master.

With his Bachelor's qualification, Hobbys was allowed to lecture on the *Aphorisms* of Hippocrates, having paid twenty shillings for the privilege. He then moved on to Cambridge where he received his MD three years later. Unusually for a university graduate, Hobbys managed to avoid the requirement of taking holy orders, perhaps because he had 'spilled blood' already during his surgeon's apprenticeship, and so was able not only to continue his career in surgery but to marry as well. His patron was Richard, Duke of York, but since Hobbys only qualified as a physician in 1459 and an MD in 1462, the majority of his service to York must have occurred during his twelve-year period of practising as a surgeon because York was killed at the Battle of Wakefield in 1460. Hobbys then went on to serve York's sons in turn, Edward IV and Richard III, as the King's Physician and King's Surgeon, being well rewarded by both monarchs[25] and, evidently, proud of his years spent attending to the health problems the House of York. We know this because in his will, written in his own hand in Latin in 1488, he sets down the Latin inscription that he wants carved on his tomb, proclaiming his years of service and loyalty to the Yorkist regime.[26] In December 1483, Richard III had granted William Hobbys, as the King's Physician, £40 per year for life, the money to be collected from fines paid to the Crown in Bedford and Buckingham.[27]

Also apparent in Hobbys's case is the fact that son followed father into medical practice. I'm uncertain how often this happened in the fifteenth century, but the will of the London surgeon John Dagvile, drawn up in 1477, bequeathed his books on physic and surgery and all his surgical instruments to his son, also John and also a surgeon.[28] Dagvile says in his will that he stood as godparent to the daughter of fellow surgeon William Wetwang, bequeathing Ellen Wetwang 6s 8d, so there was obviously friendship among the surgeons of London, their fellow practitioners and apprentices.

John Dagvile also bequeaths to his son John 'all the medicynes that be in both my shoppes', suggesting that as well as practising surgery Dagvile was an apothecary. As we've seen, apothecaries were members of the Grocers' guild and nothing to do with the Barbers' Company or the Fellowship of Surgeons, so it seems that surgeons were allowed to prepare and sell medications, in addition to their main occupation. They were also well read. John Dagvile II, son of the surgeon mentioned above, bequeathed his 'grete boke callyd Guydo' to the Fellowship of Surgeons in 1487.[29] This was most likely a medical text by the Frenchman Guido de Vigerano, a book of anatomical illustrations produced around 1340.[30]

In his will of 1475–76, Richard Esty (mentioned earlier in

chapter 2) left his seven 'best' books of surgery to the Barbers of London[31] so, presumably, his collection comprised more than that number of medical books – that was a library of considerable size for a layman in the fifteenth century.

Apothecaries

As we've seen, surgeons like John Dagvile might also work as apothecaries but, otherwise, those involved in this branch of medicine can be harder to find in the records, perhaps because their details are buried under those of their overseers' guild, the Grocers' Company. Occasionally, an apothecary was brought to prominence for some reason other than his work. For example, Laurence Swattock, an apothecary from Kingston-upon-Hull, became mayor of Hull and was a witness in a court case involving the mayor of York and a merchant, arguing over who owned a cask of Gascon wine. Swattock swore on the gospels at York in 1489 that the wine belonged to the merchant, not his fellow mayor. We also learn from Swattock's will, drawn up in April 1492, that his daughter, Agnes, lived in London and that he left two copies of a book, *The Antidotarium Nicolai*, a popular book on medicines and antidotes, to his servant (he probably means his apprentice) Henry Wytrik. We know he was married as he names Jenet, his wife, as the executrix of his will.[32]

It can be difficult to distinguish apothecaries from grocers and the two crafts often overlapped; John Clerk, principal apothecary to Edward IV (1461–83), was a prominent member of the Grocers' Company.[33] In his will, written in 1479 but not sent for probate until March 1483, he refers to himself as a citizen and grocer of London without any mention of having been a royal apothecary or a medical man of any kind.[34] Only two items in the will hint at his royal and medical connections. Firstly, he currently holds some gold plate in trust for the children of Master Roger Marchall 'late phisicion of London'. Marchall was one of the king's physicians and Clerk must have been a well-respected friend and possibly an executor of Marchall's will. Secondly, Clerk bequeaths forty shillings to Thomas Babham, who had been a servant to Queen Margaret, wife of Henry VI. Clerk lived in the parish of St Stephen's in Walbrook. He makes his second wife, Katherine, the executrix of his will.

The apothecaries who attended the king came under the jurisdiction of the royal office of the Great Spicery and the Confectionary, so close was their involvement with food products. It is these apothecaries in royal service who are easiest to identify.

Philip of Gloucester appears in the records in 1256 when he, Robert de Montpellier and Peter de Stanes, all of whom, despite their surnames, were apothecaries of London, were granted a pardon by King Henry III for having caused the death of Robert de Langele. Unfortunately, the records don't tell us how Langele died; were the four men involved in a fight or an accident? Or might his death have been caused by a medicine made up by the apothecaries? Some of the ingredients which apothecaries might add to their concoctions could have been lethal in the wrong dosage, like this medieval anaesthetic called 'dwale':

> To make a drink that men call dwale, to make a man sleep during an operation. Take the gall of a boar, three spoonfuls of the juice of hemlock and three spoonfuls of wild bryony, lettuce, opium poppy, henbane and vinegar. Mix them well together and then let the man sit by a good fire and make him drink of the potion until he falls asleep. Then he may safely be operated upon.[35]

Hemlock, opium and henbane can all put a patient to sleep – permanently. The dosage would have been a matter of guesswork because, although the ingredients would be carefully weighed and measured, there was no way to tell the strength of the active compounds. Plant samples can vary according to the age of the plant when it was gathered, where it was grown, whether leaves, stems, roots, flowers, etc. are used, how long it has stood on the shelf and under what conditions it was stored. Without knowing the strength of the medicine, the only safeguard was the bryony, a powerful laxative that hurried the mixture through and out of the body before it poisoned the patient. Perhaps Robert de Langele had suffered an unfortunate overdose of dwale or some other potion.

Nevertheless, King Henry trusted Philip of Gloucester to supply him with an assortment of medicines, many of which sound more like sweets. Philip was required to deliver 7½ pounds weight of diapenidion, a confection made from sugar, barley water and egg whites, drawn out into fine strands, along with syrups and electuaries, these last being made with honey. King Edward I (1272–1307) in 1300–01 ordered electuaries for his family to the incredible weight of 1,092 pounds.[36] Wisely, the apothecaries thought their royal patients were more likely to take their medicines as prescribed if they tasted nice, or if a sweet was given as a reward after swallowing down a less pleasant dose. Some sweets we still enjoy today were originally medicines. Liquorice sweets could be used for many ailments, from quieting an upset stomach to soothing a chesty cough. Turkish delight was a Middle Eastern medical product, the soft mixture of sugar and rose syrup being a traditional treatment for sore throats which became popular in the West probably when it was brought home by the returning crusaders. The modern Arabic name for the sweet is *rāḥat al-hulqūm*, which means 'comfort of the throat', a reminder of its original purpose.

King Edward I worked his apothecaries rather hard. Richard de Montpellier was a London spice merchant and both he and his brother, Henry, served Edward as royal apothecaries. The brothers accompanied the king to Gascony – then part of the territories of the English king as Duke of Aquitaine in France – in 1286, being

71

signed up for a year's service. In 1306, the now elderly Edward became ill at Winchester, having a problem with painful legs. Despite being prescribed ointment for his legs made from aloes and balsam and 'drying agents', there was little improvement and the king had to be carried around the country in a litter or a carriage, no longer able to ride a horse. Nevertheless, that summer Edward was determined to continue making war on the Scots, but made certain that his favourite apothecary went too, in case he needed more medications. By the time the royal party reached Hexham in Northumberland in early September the king was suffering from dysentery, and Richard of Montpellier was hastily sent all the way back to London to collect twenty-seven types of medical applications as prescribed by Edward's physician, Master Nicholas de Tyngewyke.

The list included 282 pounds weight of electuaries at 1s per pound, 106 pounds weight of 'white powder' at 2s per pound, medicinal wine, bath oils, ointments, a plaster for the king's neck and a specific honey electuary that also contained ambergris, musk, crushed pearls and gemstones, gold and silver. The medical bill came to a staggering £129 16s 4d plus another £20 to pay Richard's expenses, travelling to London and hiring five extra horses to carry all the purchases back north to rejoin the king at Carlisle. At least the treatments worked. Edward's health improved for a while, but neither his physician nor his apothecary, nor the old king himself, could fend off death for much longer. Edward died of a renewed bout of dysentery the following summer on 7 July 1307.

So now that we have some idea about how the medieval medical profession acquired its knowledge from ancient sources and how it was organised – somewhat chaotically – how did a physician, a surgeon or an apothecary set about diagnosing a patient's problems? What methods would he use?

4

DIAGNOSING THE PROBLEM

> And yit ther is another craft that toucheth the clergie,
> That ben false fisiciens that helpen men to die;
> He wole wagge [shake] his urine in a vessel of glaz,
> And swereth that he is sekere than evere yit he was ...
> *The Political Songs of England, c.* 1400

When a medieval person felt unwell, most probably one of the first things they did was to try to determine the cause. Had they recently committed a sin for which God might be punishing them by making them suffer? If their conscience was disturbed by some recent unworthy indiscretion, then making a confession to a priest, followed by contrition, penance and absolution might do the trick. If their conscience was untroubled by any sin or the services of the priest hadn't solved the problem, then maybe it was something they'd eaten or perhaps they had breathed in those 'bad airs' from the local latrines or tanneries – the latter being famous for their stench because things like stale human urine and dogs' excrement were used as part of the process to tan the leather. Like us today, those who felt off-colour might use some tried and trusted family remedy: a 'simple' maybe, made from a single herb, or perhaps an amulet or charm passed down through the generations which had proved effective in the past.

If self-medication failed, then it might be time to dig into the purse and resort to paying for professional help. The patient could choose to go to a physician, a surgeon or an apothecary. The choice might be down to who was available locally. Physicians were expensive so usually operated in the bigger towns and cities, where there were sufficient wealthy customers to keep them in business. It is estimated that in the City of York in 1381, with 7,500 inhabitants, there was only one physician and eight barber-surgeons, so clearly not everyone who fell ill could call on a qualified practitioner. Surgeons, often doubling as barbers, could make a living more easily, so a small town might well boast a surgeon or two. Apothecaries were more numerous, but only in the city would it be worthwhile for them to stock the more expensive items like dragon's blood, Venice treacle, perfumed sugars and exotic spices. A village apothecary would probably sell mainly homegrown herbs. At the lowest point on the scale and cheapest to consult would be the local wise woman, who gathered herbs in season from the woodlands, fields and hedgerows, storing, preserving and preparing them as needed. She might accept a few eggs or the mending of a broken window shutter as payment in kind for her services.

Whomever the patient consulted, the practitioner's first step would be to diagnose the problem. Talking to the patient would seem to be a good place to start, asking him how he felt, where it hurt, how long he'd had the problem, what his general state of health was like otherwise, etc. Having heard the patient's account of his ailment, the next might be to listen to the sounds his body made: the gurgles, coughing, creaking, rumbling and croaking, all useful indicators for doctors. This method is known as auscultation – listening to sounds within the body – and dates back to ancient times. The Hippocratic writings describe 'succussion' as shaking a patient to hear the splashing noises within his chest, which sounds rather unpleasant. Percussion is still carried out by doctors today: tapping the chest wall with a finger and listening with the ear for reverberations. The medieval doctor didn't have that useful tool, the stethoscope, which was invented in 1816 by René Théophile Hyacinthe Laennec (1781–1826) and transformed the way physicians detected abnormalities of the heart and chest and meant he could hear what was going on inside, while keeping a safe distance from the patient.

A good medical professional would have made use of all his senses in diagnosing the problem. Seeing and identifying the visual signs of ill health would have begun the moment the patient walked through the door or at the first sight of him in bed. A sharp eye would spot and diagnose any peculiarities, from rashes, blotches, pimples, pustules, running sores and ulcers to changes in skin colour, urine and stools, to signs of infection on the tongue, in the throat, eyes, ears, nose or discharges from any orifice of the body. If the patient looked ill that was a firm starting point for making a diagnosis.

From the patient's complexion and general demeanour, his likely dominant humour would be quite obvious to a well-trained physician, surgeon or apothecary and this had to be taken into account in the diagnosis. For example, an elderly patient, especially a female, was likely to be of a phlegmatic disposition naturally, so looking pale and weary was probably her normal condition. Therefore, if she looked flushed and frantic, it was a far more serious matter than in the case of a young man, whose natural temperament was sanguine, with red cheeks and boundless energy.

The sense of touch was used too – feeling the pulse is a practice going back at least to the time of the ancient Greeks – and physicians would take note of the regularity or abnormality of the sick patient's pulse. Taking the pulse remains a hallmark of the medical profession. Touching the patient's forehead (prior to the invention of the clinical thermometer in 1714) was, and is still, used to detect fever. Feeling for lumps and bumps was a classic way of spotting abnormalities and discovering the site of pain, but too much touching was often considered indelicate and feeling beneath the clothes was definitely undignified for a genteel physician.

The use of the senses of smell and taste as means of detecting illness might seem more unusual to us today, but the medieval practitioner wouldn't have hesitated. One of the standard ways of checking for disease was to sniff the patient's urine, stools, perspiration or breath. Unpleasant body odours, fetid breath, pus-filled sores, stinky stools and vomit might be vital in understanding the illness and doctors' case notes usually contained detailed descriptions of their patients' smells. According to Dobson, the smell of freshly baked bread from the skin or breath suggested typhoid, the smell of sweaty sheep was associated with smallpox and the odour of plucked feathers was linked with measles.[1] Tasting urine was another possibility and we know today that sweet, sugary urine is a symptom of diabetes.

An Egyptian papyrus of around 1550 BC mentions a rare disease that caused the patient to lose weight rapidly and urinate frequently. This is thought to be the first reference to diabetes.[2] The disease was first given its name by the Greek physician Aretaeus of Cappoadocia (AD 30–90) who wrote of a sickness with symptoms such as constant thirst (polydipsia), excessive urination (polyuria) and weight loss. He called the condition 'diabetes', meaning 'a flowing through'. Diabetes was a death sentence in ancient times, but Hippocrates doesn't mention it, maybe because he was certain it was incurable and a wise physician would avoid attempting any treatment. Although Aretaeus did attempt to treat it, he notes the prognosis was very poor. He wrote that 'life [with diabetes] is short, disgusting and painful'. Later, Galen recorded the rare condition and theorised that it was an affliction of the kidneys. After this, diabetes is hardly mentioned and seems to have been not only a bit of a mystery but incredibly rare during the

Middle Ages. However, Avicenna (980–1037), a famous Persian physician whose work *The Canon of Medicine* was widely read by medieval medical students, described in detail the complications of the disease, the 'abnormal appetite and the collapse of sexual functions' and how it progressed. Like Aretaeus before him, Avicenna recognised a primary (type 1) and secondary (type 2) diabetes, describing diabetes insipidus very precisely for the first time. He also described diabetic gangrene and treated diabetes using a mixture of lupin, fenugreek and zedoary seeds. This preparation considerably reduces the excretion of sugar and is a treatment still prescribed today.[3] Because it could be diagnosed by tasting the urine and finding it to be sweet, diabetes was given a second name, *mellitus*, meaning 'honey' in Latin.

Uroscopy and Urine Charts

The urine flask, sometimes called a 'Jordan' because it held the 'waters of Jordan', a medieval euphemism for 'pee', was the physician's favourite diagnostic tool, so much so that it became the badge of his profession. St Cosmas is usually pictured grasping a glass flask in his hand, his symbol as the patron saint of physicians, holding it to the light to check the colour and clarity of the urine sample. Physicians knew that the exact colour and any sign of cloudiness indicated the patient's state of health and the nature of his illness. Wealthy patients regularly sent a sample to be checked out, to make sure they weren't going down with something nasty. For example, if the urine was too pale, it was a sign of too much phlegm in the body. According to the French doctor, Guy de Chauliac,

A doctor should be willing to learn, be sober and modest, charming, hard-working and intelligent. He should care for rich and poor alike for medicine is required by all. If payment is offered he should accept it; but if it isn't offered, he shouldn't demand it. Whatever he learns of the patient during treatment must remain secret.

Fresh urine, straight from the patient, would be warm, so it was necessary for it to stay warm for proper evaluation. When the urine cools, the bubbles in it change and some disappear, particles and impurities sink to the bottom, making them more difficult to see. The urine itself would thicken, leading to the possibility of a false diagnosis. For these reasons, doctors usually inspected the urine quickly, but there were some physicians who reckoned they could diagnose the patient's illness from the urine alone without ever seeing the sick person. In this case, the fee was less and if the patient had some contagion, it was safer for the doctor to diagnose at a distance, but the urine would have been cold by the time they received the sample.

To help with this method of diagnosis, called 'uroscopy', every medical man or woman would have had a colour chart to compare to the urine sample, with colours ranging from palest yellow, through shades of green, brown and orange, to the rather scary possibilities of red, purple, blue and even black – if the urine was this colour, the illness was terminal, no treatment would be attempted and a priest summoned immediately. According to the medical handbook known as MS 8004, at the Wellcome Library, if the unfortunate patient's urine be 'as inke', then he is suffering from the quartaine fever and black jaundice and the result will be 'deth in schorte tyme'.[4] I have been intrigued by these colour charts. Was there an accepted standard chart by which all the other numerous versions were judged? Was the fact that just about all medieval glass – unless stained some other colour for decorative purposes – had a definite greenish tinge to it taken into account in these colour charts? Otherwise, the diagnosis could have been skewed.

On the subject of glass and spectacles – a necessary aid to many a learned physician, I suspect – colourless lead crystal glass was invented by the Englishman George Ravenscroft in 1674, so prior to that date things like spectacles (for aiding long-sighted people to read, etc.), prisms and lenses were usually made of polished rock crystal. The English bishop Robert Grosseteste wrote a treatise between 1220 and 1235 called *De iride* (*On the Rainbow*) in which he mentions using optics to 'read the smallest letters at incredible distances'. A few years later, in 1262, the English friar-philosopher Roger Bacon wrote in his *Opus Majus*,

> If anyone examines letters or other minute objects through the medium of crystal or glass or other transparent substance, if it be shaped like the lesser segment of a sphere, with the convex side toward the eye, he will see the letters far better and they will seem larger to him. For this reason such an instrument is useful to all persons and to those with weak eyes for they can see any letter, however small, if magnified enough.[5]

The first reading glasses are believed to have been invented in Italy in the 1280s. In 1289, an Italian, di Popozo, wrote, 'I am so debilitated by age that without the glasses known as spectacles, I would no longer be able to read or write. These have recently been invented for the benefit of poor old people whose sight has become weak.'[6]

So it seems that the first spectacles were made between 1268 and 1289. In 1306 a monk of Pisa delivered a sermon in which he said, 'It is not yet twenty years since the art of making spectacles, one of the most useful arts on earth, was discovered. I, myself, have seen and conversed with the man who made them first.'[7] Unfortunately for history, the monk didn't name the inventor of spectacles.

Returning to urine analysis, we may never know the answer to the question of colour in the glass itself, but the charts certainly brighten up the medical treatises of the time. The glass also needed to be of an even thickness throughout the urine flask. If the top was of thinner glass than the body of the flask, then any impurities in the sample might have looked different from the top and bottom, despite being the same. Uneven glass could act as a magnifier, enlarging any bits floating in the sample and so distort the diagnosis. Since identifying the colour of the urine was essential for a proper diagnosis, the lighting was crucial and daylight or candlelight were really the only options, complicating the issue still further. In strong sunlight the urine would seem too bright, but in poor light the true colour and any floating impurities would be impossible to see clearly. So the physicians' handbooks usually instructed that the urine should be examined in both conditions and the doctor must use his best judgement to make a diagnosis.

Signs of jaundice, which include the yellow discoloration of the whites of the eyes, skin, and mucous membranes, are symptoms of various diseases of the liver, such as hepatitis, that affect the processing of bile. If the urine had a brownish tint then the patient probably had jaundice. The kidneys filter waste products, especially urea, from the blood and excrete them, along with water, as urine. If the kidneys weren't working properly, were infected or damaged, the urine might appear red and/or foamy and the patient would be diagnosed as most likely suffering from kidney disease. MS 8004 tells the physician that the most healthy colour for a urine sample is 'Urine Citrine colourd lyke to a mellow appyll ... is the Uryn laudable'[8].

Other Visual Diagnoses

In July 1468, William Hattecliffe, Roger Marchall (the king's physicians we met earlier) and a colleague had their professional expertise called upon in the case of Joanna Nightingale of Brentwood in Essex. Joanna's family and neighbours believed that the unfortunate woman was suffering from leprosy and, if this was the case, she ought to withdraw from public life of any kind and retire to a leper hospital. All her goods would be forfeit and, under the law, she would be regarded as having died, but Joanna refused to go quietly, insisting she was not a leper. The sheriff was informed and summoned 'discreet men of the county who have the best knowledge of Joanna's person and of the disease', that they might make a proper diagnosis, which would be binding on Joanna and determine her fate.

Joanna was probably a widow and her family may have been a bit too eager for their inheritance. Short of hastening her end, having her condemned as a leper would produce the same result, but Joanna refused to be bullied. Before the sheriff could summon those 'discreet men', Joanna took her case to the Chancery court in London, so it seems she was wealthy enough to pay for expensive lawyers. She managed to arrange for an official judgement to be made by three of King Edward IV's personal physicians.

William Hattecliffe, Roger Marchall and Dominic de Sergio, the most distinguished physicians in England, examined Joanna thoroughly, touching her with great care, searching for signs of the dreaded disease. This was no cursory quick look, but a systematic assessment. Leprosy was determined by the presence of twenty-five 'official' common symptoms and the patient had to show at least half of them to be declared leprous. The physicians pronounced that Joanna wasn't showing enough symptoms, although there were some. However, a more detailed investigation followed based on the 'forty signs associated with the four different humoral types' (sanguine, melancholic, choleric or phlegmatic) and in this case Joanna showed no signs of the disease at all. Hattecliffe and his colleagues announced, 'And this is enough to free her from suspicion, since nobody can suffer from the disease unless they are afflicted by the greater part of these symptoms.' Their findings were made official, being noted down in Latin, and Joanna was free to return to Brentwood and resume her life.[9]

She must have been so relieved, but we can only guess at the responses of her family and neighbours. Were they still doubtful and avoided her for fear of contagion, or merely disappointed that there was to be no quick route to inheritance? I can only hope Joanna had some enjoyment out of the rest of her days, but she disappears from the record after her experiences with the king's physicians.

Phlebotomy and Blood Testing

Phlebotomy was both a method of diagnosis and a popular medical treatment throughout the Middle Ages. It continued to be a recognised and respected treatment until much later, being continued into the nineteenth century. Letting blood was thought to be a preventive, to keep you from becoming ill by keeping the body in balance. The procedure involved cutting a vein with a fleam (scalpel) and draining the blood into a bowl until the patient felt faint. At this point it was reckoned all the 'bad' blood had been removed. According to one medieval medical handbook,

> Bleeding clears the mind, strengthens the memory, cleanses the guts, sharpens the hearing, curbs tears, promotes digestion, produces a musical voice, dispels sleepiness, drives away anxiety, feeds the blood and rids it of poisonous matter and gives long life, cures pain, fevers and various sicknesses and makes urine clear and clean.[10]

With such wonderful benefits, no wonder the practice continued for centuries!

Medical instruction books often had illustrations of 'Vein Men'. These were diagrams, sometimes brightly coloured, that showed which veins the blood should be taken from, depending on the ailment suspected or being treated. The choice of vein to be bled, according to these diagrams, doesn't always sound logical: for heart problems a vein on the forehead should be cut, for neckache a vein in the ankle and for trouble with the spleen an incision should be made in the wrist. If bleeding was carried out until the patient fainted – and this was quite usual – then he had lost more than a litre of blood, which was collected in a bowl for examination. There was also the question of whether to bleed from a vein, which was usually the case, or from an artery. Arteriotomy was far more dangerous because it meant a deeper incision and the blood would spurt out. The procedure was extremely difficult to control and the blood took longer to clot, so arteries were cut only rarely. Another consideration, argued over by physicians since Galen's time, was whether to bleed the patient from close to the problem area, on the same side of the body (called 'derivation') to remove the bad blood, or from the opposite side of the body (known as 'revulsion') to draw the bad blood away and encourage good blood to flow towards the afflicted site. Both methods were practised, individual physicians tending to favour prescribing one or the other.

Whatever site was selected, the bloodletting equipment included fleams (scalpels), bleeding-bowls, cups for 'cupping', and live leeches. We may shudder at the thought, but leeches were probably the least painful method of bleeding. The leech would be attached to the appropriate vein, according to the Vein Man chart. Leech saliva is an incredible cocktail of active ingredients. It contains an anticoagulant which prevents the blood clotting, otherwise the leech would choke, but it also has anaesthetic and antibiotic properties. In the natural world, these extra assets are for the leech's benefit; the anaesthetic means the host – the animal or human from whom the leech is sucking its liquid lunch – doesn't feel anything, so it doesn't try to dislodge its uninvited guest and may not even be aware of it. The antibiotic kills off the bacteria in the host's blood, so the leech doesn't become infected with any ailment afflicting the host. Modern medicine is currently putting leeches to good use. In the past, if you accidentally chopped off a finger it was possible to surgically sew it back on, but long-term recovery was a poor prospect.

Although modern micro-surgical techniques can reattach arteries, veins and other tissues, it just isn't possible to reconnect the blood capillaries. Capillaries are finer than cobwebs, but it is within them that blood nutrients and oxygen are exchanged for waste matter and carbon dioxide in the surrounding tissue. Without this exchange, the tissues will die. However, capillaries can regrow themselves within a matter of days, if the tissues can be kept healthy until then. This is where the leeches come in: they are attached to the site of healing and feed on the blood that accumulates there. As one leech falls off, having taken its fill, a new one replaces it. The process can take anything from twenty minutes to an hour. What they are doing, quite unintentionally, is completing the circulation cycle, removing the blood that would otherwise be flowing from the capillaries, back into the veins and away, allowing fresh, oxygenated blood to come into the recovering tissues to keep them healthy while they repair. After a few days, the leeches are no longer needed as the circulation is restored through the new capillaries.

The anticoagulants in leech saliva may have applications in future treatments to prevent blood clots (thromboses), heart attacks and strokes, or after heart valve replacement surgery, where warfarin is used at present. Warfarin can be a danger in itself and lethal if taken in conjunction with certain other commonly used drugs, so a safer alternative would be welcome and leeches may provide it. Other ingredients in the leech-saliva cocktail are the subjects of continuing medical research. The local anaesthetics have possibilities as painkillers as well as applications for minor surgery. The antibiotic elements may be even more important as the urgent search goes on for some means of conquering bacteria, which are evolving resistance to available antibiotics at an ever-increasing rate. The saliva contains about fifty different chemical compounds that have been identified, many of them still to be investigated as to their possible uses in modern medicine.

To return to bloodletting, if the patient was thought unable to withstand the rigors of cutting a vein with a fleam, or the application of leeches, there was a third alternative. Cupping, as it was called, was believed to be less traumatic for the patient, so this method was recommended for use on children, pregnant women, the elderly and anyone who seemed particularly frail. Despite such recommendations, cupping sounds a most unpleasant process. Before cupping, the skin would be 'scarified' with an instrument that had a series of tiny blades, or pins, which pierced the skin. A glass cup was heated and held against the scarified skin. As the hot air in the cup cooled, the air pressure decreased, creating a partial vacuum, attaching the cup to the skin and 'sucking' out the blood. A whole series of cups could be used at once on different parts of the patient's body in the same treatment session, so he would be sore all over afterwards.

Whatever method of phlebotomy was chosen, the intention was to remove the excess of blood – the plethora – because a surplus of blood, clogging up the body, was the most common cause of illness. The medieval physician had no idea that blood circulated; that was a mystery to him. Instead, he believed that blood was made in the liver, flowed out and was used up in the tissues as nourishment. This nourishment came directly from food and drink consumed by the patient, which was the reason why the correct diet was so important in both treating the sick and maintaining good health in those who were well. If the liver made too much, or the body didn't consume enough blood, the system became unbalanced and the body fell sick.

Taking the Pulse

Another aid in determining what ailed the patient was to take his pulse. Quite a simple procedure, you might think, but in the Middle Ages, before clocks and watches, how could you time the pulse? Instead, physicians described the pulse as moving 'like a snail or an ant' or even 'a gazelle' – always supposing they knew what a gazelle was. These descriptions had been set down by the Roman doctor Galen, who probably knew a bit about gazelles from his time in Africa, but whether an English physician would realise a gazelle was a lively creature that leapt and bounded about is impossible to say. Nevertheless, the descriptions remained and crop up in many medieval medical texts as guidelines. How a pulse described as 'like a gazelle' was then related to the symptoms of a particular ailment must have been a tricky question, even for a university-trained physician.

The Greek medical texts, from which Galen had taken much of his basic information and which were available to medieval scholars, went into a great deal of detail about the pulse. Every individual, even in the best of health, would have had a unique pulse type, depending on his basic temperament. According to Greek medicine, a pulse that slithers like a snake denotes that the individual is of a melancholic temperament. The snake or serpentine pulse is firm, clearly defined and often thin, indicating dryness. It also tends to be fast and rather weak from an excess of nervous energy. If the individual has a choleric temperament, his normal, healthy pulse will be like a frog, forceful and bounding, rather rapid but not so fast, surprisingly, as a serpentine pulse. The pulse of a phlegmatic individual will glide smoothly as a swan, slow, soft and deep. Since the sanguine temperament is the most balanced of all, the sanguine pulse is moderate, undulating freely like a playful dolphin. The pulse of a sanguine individual combines the flowing smoothness and fluidity (moist quality) of the phlegmatic swan with the energy and exuberance (hot quality) of the choleric frog, so it is relaxed and supple.[11]

When a patient became unwell, his normal pulse would change because a different humour was now in excess, depending on which ailment he was suffering from. The four elemental qualities – hot, cold, moist and dry – each produced a basic, identifiable type of pulse. A hot quality was indicated by a rapid pulse or one that was forceful and bounding. A cold quality was indicated by a slow, 'deep' pulse. A weak pulse could also be a sign of cold, since it indicated a lack of energy. Acute cold, as in catching a cold or a chill, could constrict the pulse, or a longstanding cold distemper might produce a tense pulse.

Excessive moisture was indicated by a soft or soggy pulse, caused by a superfluity of blood and/or other humours. A wet, slippery pulse was often found in pregnant women who needed increased amounts of the moist, flourishing phlegmatic and sanguine humours to nourish their growing foetus. The pulsations caused by too much moisture were described as 'seeming to roll out from under your fingers like pearls in a bowl'. Too dry a quality was indicated by a clearly defined pulse which was firm but sometimes thin and rough because of a deficiency of moist flourishing humours, contrary to the smoothness of the slippery pulse. A choppy pulse was often associated with a dry temperament, but if it was also thin, it denoted a deficiency of blood and phlegm, or a systemic stagnation of the blood. An excess of cold quality was indicated by a slow, weak pulse, tense or constricted, thin and clearly defined. Despite the obvious complexity and problems in actually describing the pulse, an experienced physician could tell a strong, steady rhythm from a weak, faltering one, or one that raced. The usual standard by which he judged it was by comparing the patient's pulse to his own, taking that as being normal.

So, by one means or another, or maybe a combination of methods, the medical practitioner – physician, surgeon or apothecary – had diagnosed the patient's problems, but before any form of treatment could begin, the prognosis for the ailment had to be worked out. Was it worth treating the patient or was he certain to die, whatever was done? The art of prognosis could amount to fortune telling or foreseeing the future, but how was this done in the field of medicine?

5

PROGNOSIS – FORETELLING WHETHER THE PATIENT WILL LIVE OR DIE

Therefore, the general rule should be never to proceed in any disease unless one has first prognosticated. Indeed, prognostication is not to be neglected.

Bernard de Gordon, Montpellier (*fl.* 1270–1330)

Prognosis today refers to the likely course of a disease. If we catch a cold, we know that the first sniffles will get worse before our body is able to do battle and fight it off, the whole process taking about ten days, barring further complications such as catarrh or a chest infection. In the Hippocratic writings it says, 'I believe that it is an excellent thing for a physician to practise forecasting. He will carry out the treatment best if he knows beforehand from the present symptoms what will take place later.' Medieval doctors understood the way many common diseases progressed, developing, worsening until a crisis was reached. At this point, either the patient won the fight and began to recover or else he started to slip away. Hippocrates had explained all this, as well as the possibilities of remission or relapse.[1]

But a number of factors made prognosis even more important in medieval times, not least the Church's insistence that the soul was what really mattered and the body was merely its earthly container. If the prognosis was bad and the patient sure to die, whatever the physician or surgeon did in an attempt to save him, it was far better, said the Church, for the medical men to step back and let the priest do his job of preparing the soul for departure to the next life. It would also give the patient time to write his will, set his affairs in order and prepare for death. The law also had a say in the matter – if the patient was given medical treatment but became worse, or even died, there was always the possibility of the physician or surgeon being prosecuted by the patient, his family, or even his fellow professionals, if they thought the doctor had been negligent or made mistakes – litigation for malpractice wasn't unknown.

Finally, there was the doctor's own reputation to consider. If he took on a hopeless case, with the patient either sick or injured beyond saving, it hardly helped his professional standing if he had to add another death to his list. Such a failure would not encourage more patients to his door and he had a living to make. Obviously, the best patient was one with a good chance of recovery and medical handbooks advised that patients unlikely to recover should be avoided at all costs and not treated at all. However, if the patient probably was going to get better, the physician had everything to gain by giving the correct diagnosis and treatment that would bring about the return to good health. Every doctor must have realised that if he took on a very poorly patient who actually recovered after all, this would do wonders for his reputation and expand his practice. The problem was how the medical profession – without X-rays, MRI scanners or even stethoscopes – could tell whether a patient looked worse than was in fact the case, or if one who appeared a bit under the weather might not rapidly deteriorate and die.

With so much at stake, physicians, surgeons and apothecaries resorted to techniques that we would think of as strange and hardly to be associated with medicine at all: divination, astrology and even magic.

Astrology, Horoscopes and 'Zodiac Men'

At university, physicians were trained in the art of drawing up horoscopes – your health was written in the stars. Everyone would have a natal chart based upon the positions of the planets at the exact moment of their birth and each body part was affected by one of the signs of the Zodiac. As an aid to remembering which body part was influenced by a particular sign, medical handbooks often included a 'Zodiac Man' – a drawing of a naked man with the signs of the Zodiac strategically placed to show which area each dominated, or else draped with scrolls bearing the names of the signs. These images were frequently in full colour and really brightened up a dull old textbook.

The Zodiac Man in MS 8004 is a pen drawing festooned with scrolls against a vivid red ground, with blue borders on either side and at the top, surrounded by a gold frame. It seems to have been the page most frequently referred to in the whole manuscript; it is certainly the most well-worn and rubbed, so it got a great deal of use. According to these Zodiac Men, Aries, for example, had domination over the head. When the moon – the most significant planet in astrological medicine, influencing the bodily humours just as it caused the tides to ebb and flow – was in the house of Aries, it was not only dangerous, but potentially fatal to treat the head in any way. This included washing, combing, shaving, applying any medication to it, and certainly no blood was to be taken from it, especially by inducing a nosebleed to purge the brain.[2] Cases were brought to the law courts against physicians and surgeons who failed to take into account the moon's position when treating a patient, if the outcome wasn't good, as we'll see in chapter 8.

Alongside the Zodiac Man, it was useful to have some means of quickly looking up the phase of the moon and the position of the sun in a particular zodiacal house (i.e. the day's date). The volvelle was invented for exactly this purpose; it was a series of concentric discs of parchment on which the physician could dial up the date, set the phase of the moon disc and see which sign of the Zodiac it pointed to. If it was Pisces, then no treatment could be applied to the feet; if it was Leo, nothing could be done to the chest; and so on. The Guild Book of the Barber-Surgeons of York,[3] dated to 1486, has both a volvelle (f.51r) – described as 'a circular zodiacal lunar scheme with a rotary disc and pointer, representing the sun' – and a Zodiac Man (f.50v) or *homo signorius* (Sign Man), as the scribe called it. As well as the illustrated disc, the volvelle page is further decorated in the top corners with images of John the Baptist and St John the Evangelist, and in the lower corners with the images of St Cosmas the physician with his urine flask, and St Damian the surgeon with his box of medicinal powders – the four patron saints of the guild. The book also contains a drawing of the head of Christ surrounded by personifications of the four humours (f.51v). The scrolls that loop across this page tell how the humours relate to the complexions of man and to the four elements. The figures themselves are a fascinating window onto late fifteenth-century male fashion, from melancholic man's disreputably short doublet, striped hose and large purse, to sanguine man's more modest doublet and purse of middling size, to the red-haired (i.e. ill-tempered), choleric man in his knee-length gown and, finally, the elderly phlegmatic man who wears the longest gown and mittens to keep him warm, but is so old-fashioned with his floppy hat and pointed-toe boots.

The almanac or *vade mecum* (Latin for 'go with me'), in the form of a 'girdle-book', was invented as a means of carrying around all this necessary information. These little books were constructed from sheets of parchment pages stitched together, each folded to a handy size within a cover, small enough to hang from the practitioner's girdle or belt. The almanac would contain the phases of the moon, a Vein Man, maybe a volvelle and a Zodiac Man and perhaps a chart of the four humours and any other charts which might assist in diagnosing the patient's problem and making the appropriate prognostication. A precious little almanac known as MS 40, in the Wellcome Library in London, is a fine example, but is now too fragile to be handled although a replica copy has been promised. It has seven sheets of vellum, each folded in two and then into three, forming a booklet of fourteen centimetres by five centimetres in a soft cover with a tag, so it could be hung from a belt. The text and drawings are in red and black ink with blue initials and two detailed diagrams, one of a Vein Man and the other of a Zodiac Man, both carefully drawn. It includes an illustrated list of lunar eclipses dating from 1461 to 1481, with '1463' inscribed on the cover in fifteenth-century handwriting.[4]

We saw in chapter 1 that medieval scholars believed a particular conjunction of the stars and planets was to blame for the epidemic of plague which ravaged Europe in 1348–50. Philip VI of France asked the medical experts at the University of Paris to look into the causes of the outbreak in October 1348. After consulting their books and star charts, the experts informed the king that no human agent was to blame; no wells had been poisoned, as had been feared. The fatal moment had occurred three years earlier, at one o'clock in the afternoon on 25 March 1345. The report explained how Mars, Jupiter and Saturn had all come together at that time in the house of Aquarius. The combination of Jupiter and Saturn was destined to cause 'the death of peoples and the depopulation of kingdoms'. Jupiter – a warm, humid planet – and Mars – a hot, dry planet – together in the warm, humid sign of Aquarius, caused so much heat that evil vapours were drawn up from the earth and water. Then the dry heat of Mars set the vapours on fire with lightning bolts and strange lights in the sky. Mars turned its 'evil aspect' towards Jupiter and remained at its most malevolent from October 1347 until May 1348.[5] A physician from Montpellier pointed out that Saturn had looked on Mars with an evil aspect too, so no wonder the worst befell.

Occasionally, the astrologers even got their predictions right. The London astrologer Richard Trewythian foretold that the people of Kent would make war on London Bridge at the beginning of July 1450.[6] He was right. Jack Cade's Kentish rebels fought a battle on the bridge and managed to cross the Thames into the City of London on the night of 4 July.

We might scoff at such ideas but, at the time, this was the cutting edge of science and to be taken very seriously indeed. Because astrology had provided the only explanation for the plague epidemic, the subject became more important than ever before, with specialist colleges of astrology being founded. Charles V of France had such a college set up in Paris, providing it with a fine library and a collection of astrological instruments.[7] It was also a kind of insurance policy for the physician, knowing his patient's fate was predetermined in the stars and, therefore, his life or death was beyond earthly control.

To help a physician to see how a patient's birth sign would affect his humoral temperament, a medical handbook often had a chart of some description to guide him. This version is found in a number of manuscripts, including MS 8004:

Aries	Leo	Sagittarius	Fire	East	Choleric	Hot & dry
Cancer	Scorpio	Pisces	Water	North	Phlegmatic	Cold & moist
Taurus	Virgo	Capricorn	Earth	South	Melancholic	Cold & dry
Gemini	Libra	Aquarius	Air	West	Sanguine	Hot & moist

Drawing up the patient's natal horoscope to work out the prognosis of his ailment could be a problem in the days before birth registration and accurate clocks. It even mattered what the phase of the moon happened to be at the time. A child born on the fifth day of the moon's cycle might well become a lunatic;[8]

a baby born on the twelfth day would be especially pious.[9] But some people wouldn't have known the exact moment of their birth and maybe not even the date, yet a few minutes could make a difference to their planetary aspect. However, all was not lost. Instead of using the patient's horoscope to learn whether he was to die shortly or not, the physician could draw up the horoscope of the moment when the illness began in order to predict its outcome. Even so, this could be difficult if the illness had begun with such vague symptoms that it was impossible to determine the exact moment when the sickness started. In this case, the physician could turn to a form of magical divination, using numerology – the mystical significance of numbers and their meaning.

The Spheres of Pythagoras

The spheres of Pythagoras were circular diagrams, so called because the Greek mathematician had, supposedly, invented them. However, the earliest version still in existence, in this case called 'The sphere of Life and Death', is in a manuscript known as Papyrus V of Leyden, dated to the fourth century AD and attributed to Democritus. Whoever invented these diagrams, they were a means of prophesying the future by following a number code for the letters of the patient's name – in other words, the likely outcome of the illness; whether the patient would live or die. The spheres of Pythagoras were perfect for giving the correct answer – or simply the answer the physician wanted – because he could use the patient's Christian name or surname or both together with any spelling as imaginative as he wished to give the number required.

The instructions for using the spheres, as given in MS 8004, tell the physician to count the letters in the patient's name using A=1, B=2, C=3, etc. Then add them all together, plus the number assigned to the phase of the moon on the day that the patient first fell sick. Next, divide this total by thirty as many times as possible and the remainder is the important bit. For example, if the first total came to 115, divided by thirty this gives three with a remainder of twenty-five. Look up the number twenty-five on the sphere diagram. If it is above the centre line (like an equator) then the patient will live; below the line, the prognosis is the worst: he will die.

All might not be lost even then, if the physician happened to have more than one copy of the spheres. During my research, I found versions in which, as an example, L=6 in a tenth-century sphere of Apuleius, L=21 in an eleventh-century sphere of Pythagoras and L=50 (as in the Roman numeral) in a thirteenth-century sphere. So there was every chance of getting the desired answer, one way or another. These discrepancies don't seem to have lessened the popularity of the fortune-telling devices which continued to appear in medical handbooks into the fifteenth and sixteenth centuries. Another element of prognosis which could usually be determined from these spheres but for which I can find no instructions in MS.8004, was that of the timescale: whether the patient's recovery or demise would occur rapidly or slowly or somewhere in between. It was also possible, apparently, to use them for other purposes entirely such as finding lost items, determining the best day to embark upon a new enterprise or journey,[10] even to work out the compatibility of a couple about to be wed, the success, or otherwise, of their marriage and which partner would be the first to die.

Closely linked to the use of the spheres of Pythagoras, a good physician had a thorough understanding of 'perilous days'. There were calendars available, often accredited to the Anglo-Saxon monk the Venerable Bede, which set out the good and bad days, not only for medical purposes but for any undertaking.[11] Every month had at least two 'dismal days', one during the waxing of the moon and one during its waning, when any kind of medical intervention was best avoided. It was also noted that it was especially harmful to catch a cold at any time in October, according to MS 8004. For women, the last day of December and 1 and 2 January were especially perilous, although men needed to take care at that time too and on no account was anyone to be bled on those dates because 'all the veins are then full' – of Christmas and New Year spirit, perhaps. It is a fact that alcohol thins the blood and makes bleeding from any wound more profuse and difficult to staunch, so that may be one explanation for these dates being best avoided. Like the spheres of Pythagoras, the calendar of perilous days had other uses, as in this extract from MS 8004 (I have modernised the spelling here):

Astronomers and astrologers both say that there are 29 ill days in the year in the which if any woman be wedded other[wise] they shall be departed soon or else live ever in sorrow and care together. [A]nd who so takes [a] voyage he shall never come [home] again.[12]

For any patient unfortunate enough to fall ill on a perilous day, not only was the prognosis grim but treatment of any kind would have to be delayed until a better date.

The Mysterious Caladrius Bird

A very different method of determining whether the patient would recover or die was to bring a caladrius bird to his bedside – always supposing the physician knew where to find such a creature. Within the pages of medieval bestiaries, the reader could learn of the peculiar habits of the caladrius. Bestiary books were most popular in England in the twelfth and thirteenth centuries. They were encyclopaedias about animals. Creatures both real and – to us – mythical were beautifully illustrated in these manuscripts. In MS Bodley 764, the tragelaphus (a bearded stag), 'three kinds' of lion, the manticore (which has a man's head, a lion's body and a scorpion's sting in its tail), the dragon and the unicorn are listed and described alongside the far more mundane cow, the raven, the cat, the pelican and the worm.[13]

Unlike a modern nature book, bestiaries were more concerned with the religious aspects of these creatures, assuming God had created them for man's benefit and instruction. The benefits of a cow, or even a cat as a mousecatcher, are obvious, but of what use was, say, a tiger? Tigers are, apparently, extremely vain creatures that love to admire themselves in ponds or puddles at every opportunity. Therefore, to catch a tiger, simply put a mirror in a handy spot and wait. Eventually, a passing tiger will find the mirror and gaze lovingly at his reflection for hours. Throw the net over him and the tiger is caught. The moral is that vanity will be a Christian's downfall. Bestiaries are full of similar moral tales, rather like the ancient Greek Aesop's fables, but a Christian version with lots of references to Jesus Christ.

Returning to the caladrius bird. It is usually white and looks like a cross between a seagull and a swan, depending on the illuminator's interpretation. In MS Bodley – where it is called the 'charadrius' – it is described as a river bird, entirely white without a 'speck of black' and its dung will cure poor eyesight.[14] The caladrius had close associations with Alexander the Great in the past and must have learned to appreciate good living because it now likes to make its home in royal palaces – a clue to where a physician in need might find one. Taken to a patient, if the bird will not look at the sick person, then his illness will prove fatal. However, if it looks the patient in the eye, the prognosis is excellent. The bestiaries explain that the unblemished caladrius bird is like Christ, taking the patient's sins – and the sickness they cause – upon itself, then flying away with them so that the patient can be made whole again.[15]

Throughout this chapter I have referred to physicians, rather than surgeons or apothecaries, because it was the university-trained physicians who dealt with the theories of prognosis. From my research, I get the feeling that, for the most part, surgeons and apothecaries were concerned to get on with the more practical side of medicine: treating the sick or injured. So what kinds of treatment and remedies were available to the medieval patient?

6

TREATING THE PROBLEM – FROM THE SENSIBLE TO THE UNBELIEVABLE

> Full redy hadde he his apothecaries
> To send hym drogges and his letuaries ...
> Of his diete mesurable was he,
> For it was of no superfluitee,
> But of greet norissyng and digestible.
> 'The Doctour of Phisik' from Chaucer's *Canterbury Tales*
> The General Prologue, I, lines 425–26 & 435–37

The epigraph at the head of this chapter refers to Chaucer's physician having on hand his favourite apothecaries, to make the drugs and electuaries (medicinal syrups made with honey) his patients needed, and, for his own good health, a nourishing and digestible diet was key. The importance of what you ate and drank was never underestimated by medieval medical practitioners, in fact a holistic approach to both keeping healthy and treating the sick involved not only diet, but all-round lifestyle as well. This meant a physician could talk to his patient on the most intimate subjects, even to a woman.

Before we look at how a physician might give treatment to a patient, it is worth mentioning something we've all heard of, but probably know very little about: the Hippocratic oath. There is a tradition that a great plane tree still stands on the island of Kos, in the Aegean, under which, it is said, young men were formally initiated into the art of medicine as long ago as the end of the fifth century BC. With their fellows and elders gathered around, they would take an oath, now known as the Hippocratic oath, renowned throughout the centuries for setting a high standard of professional conduct for physicians. At that time, it symbolised the spirit of the school at Kos under the leadership of Hippocrates but, despite what many people believe, it isn't a fixed and definitive statement of medical ethics, having been modified relentlessly over time. Here are some of the important points of the oath, which was sworn in the name of the god Apollo:

I will use my power to help the sick to the best of my ability and judgement; I will abstain from harming or wronging any man by it.

I will not give a fatal draught to anyone if I am asked, nor will I suggest any such thing; neither will I give a woman means to procure an abortion.

I will not abuse my position to indulge in sexual contacts with the bodies of women or men.

Whatever I see or hear, professionally or privately, which ought not to be divulged, I will keep secret and tell no one.[1]

The first point is clearly most important and as relevant today as it ever was. The second is the basis for the objections to abortion and euthanasia, and the third, sadly, is occasionally broken to the distress of patients and the loss of reputation to the profession. The fourth point is the confidentiality clause so frequently used in the plots of modern crime novels and dramas. However, the truth is that the oath has never been widely sworn by medical students or graduates; in fact, most British doctors have never even seen it, nor has the swearing of it been imposed as a condition for gaining a medical degree or going into practice. The earliest certain evidence of the oath being sworn in a university comes from 1558, and not until 1804 is there any evidence of it being sworn by newly fledged doctors.

Healthy Living Self-Help Books

For those who might have preferred not to consult a physician immediately, or couldn't afford the cost of a consultation, one possible source of instruction, a kind of medical self-help book for the layman, was the *Tacuinum Sanitatis* or 'Table of Health'. Quite a few versions of this book still exist. Most come from northern Italy originally and the text was based on an eleventh-century book written by a famous Arab physician, Ibn Butlan. He had taken his information from ancient Greek and Roman writers, covering food, drink, environments and activities and their effects on health. By the thirteenth century, the *Tacuinum* had been translated from Arabic to Latin for western readers and in the fourteenth century it was reproduced as a picturebook. This version became very popular with the Italian nobility, like the Viscontis, and beautifully illustrated copies were soon spreading across Europe.

So many subjects are covered, each with its merits and drawbacks and means of countering the latter. Some are rather obvious – such as the remedy for insomnia is sleep – while others are very sensible. For example, under the heading 'Tailor', it is noted that wool can irritate the skin, so it is advisable to line a woollen tunic with linen. This entry is interesting because it says 'the finest kind of wool comes from Flanders'. Clearly, the writer knew where the best cloth came from; what he didn't know was that the best sheep's fleece to make that cloth originated in England. Under the heading 'Robust red wine', it is noted 'it can be harmful to the liver', as we know today. However, the *Tacuinum* has the answer – to drink it with pomegranate. Here is a selection of other entries to give a flavour of the book:

70. Salted meat: The best salt meat is made from fatty animals and is good for those with phlegmatic temperaments and labourers. It should never be cooked with lentils as this combination causes terrifying dreams. 85. Crayfish: The choicest crayfish are lemon coloured and these have aphrodisiac properties. However, they can cause drowsiness which can be averted by sprinkling with almond oil. 102. Rose water: [It] should be made from the most fragrant flowers. It is good for the heart and prevents fainting, and should be taken with sugary syrup to avoid irritating the respiration. 105. Spring: The best part of spring falls in the middle of the season, when it is beneficial to all plants and animals. Bathing is advised as spring can be dangerous for dirty bodies. 114. Winter rooms: These should be heated to the temperature of the air at the end of spring in order to awaken faculties. These rooms should face north, otherwise they cause thirst and poor digestion. 125. Hunting: The ideal form of hunting is the easiest kind which thins the humours. It can dry out the body, so oiling the body while bathing is recommended.[2]

Even architecture, through the orientation of the rooms in the house, was important, as in 114 quoted above. The Chenie family of Amersham in Buckinghamshire, England, took this to extremes when they built their new manor house in 1460. Fearful of plague-ridden miasmas wafting their way from London, the house was built facing away from the city and the back walls had neither windows nor doors – although one or two small openings have been knocked through since then – to ensure that the lethal miasmas didn't blow into the rooms.

The purpose of the *Tacuinum* and other, similar treatises was to keep you in good health and medical men weren't alone in compiling this kind of guide. The fourteenth-century monk and poet John Lydgate wrote his *Treatise for Health* in verse:

> For helth of body cover for cold thy hed.
> Ete no raw mete, take gud hed ther to
> Drynke holsom wyne, feed thee on lighte bred,
> With an abbytyd [appetite] rys up from thy mete. Also
> With woman agyd [aged] have nought fleshly to do.

This poem, which continues for eighty-seven lines, was then borrowed by others. The London surgeon Richard Esty copied it into his medical handbook in 1454 and John of Burgundy used a slightly different version in 1490.[3]

King Edward IV, in 1474, issued new rules for his royal physicians, surgeons and apothecaries to follow. The duties of his physicians included using their expertise as nutritionists to work out a suitable diet for him.[4] This seems to have involved getting a dispensation from the Church so that Edward could be excused from eating fish on fast days. It is likely that the king was of a most phlegmatic disposition, i.e. he had an excess of cold, moist humours; either that or he just didn't like fish very much and, being royal, had the means of avoiding it. The physicians were also required to 'devyse' the king's medicines and keep their eyes open for any signs of disease among the courtiers, for fear they might infect the royal family. Anyone showing symptoms of leprosy or plague was to be removed from court until 'he be purged clenely' and the king should be informed immediately. For the king's son Edward, Prince of Wales, both a physician and surgeon were employed in his household and it was specified that they had to be sufficiently 'cunning' – a word that meant skilful, clever and knowledgeable and, perhaps in this case 'persuasive' as well – to see that the young prince went to bed 'joyoux and merry'.

Another sure means of warding off nasty diseases or the effects of any poison or venomous creature was to carry a snake stone at all times. These stones intrigued medieval folk, who believed they were the remains of coiled snakes turned to solid rock by God as a punishment for their evil ways. Far less of a mystery to us, they nevertheless remain fascinating – not snakes but fossilised prehistoric sea creatures; we call them ammonites.

So much for preventive medicine. However, supposing, despite everyone's best efforts, that just wasn't enough to prevent you falling ill? If you became unwell, what remedies were available? You may suppose from the title of this book that medicines went from the reasonable to the seemingly outrageous – from willow bark to dragon's blood.

Reasonable Medicines and Treatments

Some medieval remedies really did contain effective ingredients which are still in use today, or are being 'rediscovered' by current medical research. Treatments for pain and fever, going back to the time of Galen and beyond, might contain white willow bark (*Salix alba*) – a source of natural salicylic acid, similar to the active ingredient in aspirin, acetylsalicylic acid. Remedies for headache frequently contained the wildflowers betony, vervain and meadowsweet. Betony (*Stachys officinalis*) could be taken internally or applied externally, as in the recipe below. Incidentally, any plant that has *officinalis* as part of its Latin name was used in medicine in the past. Betony used to be the sovereign remedy for all maladies of the head, and its properties as a nervine (nerve tonic) are still recognised, although it is most often used in combination with other nervines.[5] One of its medieval names was 'woundwort' because it eased the pain of injuries and was believed to promote healing. It was also used to treat hysteria, palpitations, pain in the head and face, neuralgia and any other nervous problems. Today, it is still used in migraine treatments, its active ingredients being the alkaloids betonicine, stachydrine and trigonelline. Here is a fifteenth-century headache remedy that might well have worked, as the writer states at the end:

> For the migraine. Take half a dishful of barley, one handful each of betony, vervain and other herbs that are good for the head and when they be well boiled together, take them up and wrap them in a cloth and lay them to the sick head and it shall be whole. I proved it.[6]

One of the other ingredients in this remedy is vervain (*Verbena officinalis* or its modern name *Verbena hastata*) and it too is still used in modern medicine as an antidepressant and nervine. In medieval times, it was given to nursing mothers to stimulate lactation, as well as being a treatment for jaundice, gout and kidney stones, but there has been little clinical research into its possible use in modern medicine. It contains a particularly active tannin, but this has not yet been properly analysed.[7]

Vervain was worn round the neck as a charm against headaches and also against snake and other venomous bites, as well as for good luck and good eyesight. Its numerous virtues were due to the legend of its discovery on the Mount of Calvary, where it staunched the wounds of the crucified Saviour – hence it was also called the 'Herb of Grace'. When gathering vervain, the picker had to make the sign of the cross and bless the plants with a commemorative verse. It must be picked before flowering and dried promptly. In modern alternative medicine, vervain is used to treat fevers, ulcers, ophthalmia and pleurisy. As a poultice, it is good for easing headaches (as in the medieval remedy above), earache and rheumatism and in this form it colours the skin a deep red, which gave rise to the idea that it had the power of drawing the blood out. It can also be applied externally for haemorrhoids (piles).

Meadowsweet (*Filipendula ulmaria*) may well have been an ingredient in the migraine remedy above as one of the 'other herbs that are good for the head'. This plant is being re-evaluated for its medicinal properties as it also contains salicylic acid, but is less abrasive to the stomach lining than aspirin. The old Latin name for meadowsweet was *Spirea ulmaria* and the word 'aspirin' was taken from this – *a* from *acetyl* and *spirin* from *Spirea* – according to Gerald (p. 132) and Laws (p. 175). In the future, both white willow bark and meadowsweet may prove safer alternatives for patients who take aspirin daily as a cardiovascular prophylactic (a preventive medicine). The fragrant meadowsweet used to be called 'meadwort', as Geoffrey Chaucer refers to it in his *Canterbury Tales*, where it is one of the fifty ingredients in a drink called 'Save', mentioned in 'The Knight's Tale'. The flowers were often put into wine and ale, giving the drink a delicate aniseed taste, and it is still used to flavour many herb beers today. Meadowsweet was held sacred by the Druids, long ago. The garden plant *Astilbe* is the cultivated version.

A decoction of the root of meadowsweet in white wine was an excellent treatment for fevers.[8] Both the dainty spires of creamy-white flowers, which are in blossom from June to almost September, and the dark-green leaves smell delicious. The dried leaves were infused in hot water – like making tea – sweetened with honey and taken for headaches and as an anti-inflammatory for rheumatic pain. The flowers were infused similarly to treat colds, influenza, fluid retention and arthritis. Today, we know that meadowsweet also has antiseptic and diuretic properties and is good for easing the symptoms of cystitis and other urinary tract infections.[9]

Apart from its medicinal uses, meadowsweet was one of the fragrant herbs used to strew the floors of chambers, being especially popular with Queen Elizabeth I. In a way, though, this too might be considered 'medicinal', its almond-like scent banishing all those poisonous miasmas in the form of bad odours. The Tudor herbalist John Gerard (*c.* 1545–1612), writes,

The leaves and floures of Meadowsweet farre excelle all other strowing herbs for to decke up houses, to strawe in chambers, halls and banqueting-houses in the summer-time, for the smell thereof makes the heart merrie and joyful and delighteth the senses. ... It is reported that the floures boiled in wine and drunke do take away the fits of a quartaine ague and make the heart merrie. The distilled water of the floures dropped into the eies taketh away the burning and itching thereof and cleareth the sight.[10]

Meadowsweet is still a valuable medicine in the treatment of diarrhoea, especially in children and, because of its diuretic properties, is a helpful remedy for some forms of oedema (dropsy).

Having treated the patient for headache, fever and inflammation, let's now deal with his stomach problems. Anise was very popular for treating digestive problems and wind. In 1305 Edward I put a tax on it, suggesting anise was imported regularly from the Eastern Mediterranean and, according to the Royal Wardrobe Accounts, in 1480 King Edwards IV's underwear and shirts were scented with little bags of 'fustian stuffed with ireos [oris root] and anneys'.[11] Note: this wasn't star anise, which comes from the Far East and was unknown in the West in medieval times, but aniseed – not so attractive but with the same flavour and carminative properties. Here are a few fifteenth-century remedies that may well have been effective:

For fever of the stomach. Take cumin, anise, fennel-seed, red rose leaves, wormwood, mint, vinegar, sour bread, fried in a pan and made into a plaster, and lay it in a bag to the stomach lukewarm, and renew it often with vinegar.[12]

A powder for the stomach. Take powder of ginger, galingale and mint, of each equally much and use them with a quantity of wine or ale at morn and in sage at even.[13]

For sickness. Take the seed of anise, cumin, caraway, fennel, watercress and peony, each an ounce; the berries of bay, two drachms; of nutmegs, small shredded, an ounce and a half; of ginger, mace and cloves, two drachms; of liquorice as much as sufficeth to make all these sweet in a drug, which thou use morning and evening.[14]

The first recipe would certainly ease a stomach ache, cumin, anise, fennel and mint being very calming and carminative. I'm unsure what purpose was served by the red rose leaves – it may mean 'petals' – but wormwood (*Artemisis absinthium*) was used to dispel parasitic worms from the gut, so that would have helped if roundworm or tapeworm was the cause of the problem. That unfortunate king Richard III might well have felt the benefits of a dose of wormwood, since new research has shown that he suffered from roundworm (*Ascaris lumbricoides*).[15] This infection could have made him nauseous and uncomfortable, as well as causing diarrhoea. Ginger and mint, in the second recipe, are excellent for aiding digestion and easing heartburn or indigestion. In the third recipe – I'm not sure about the watercress and peony seed, or the bay berries – all the spices are known to assist digestion, to be soothing to an upset stomach and good as carminatives for getting rid of wind. Even today, ginger biscuits are recommended for mild morning sickness during pregnancy, so this remedy most probably worked.

Common wormwood had a good reputation in medicine since ancient times and the Tudor writer Thomas Tusser, in his *July's Husbandry* of 1577, instructed,

> While Wormwood hath seed get a handful or twaine
> To save against March, to make flea to refraine:
> Where chamber is sweeped and Wormwood is strowne,
> What saver is better (if physick be true)
> For places infected than Wormwood and Rue?
> It is a comfort for hart and the braine
> And therefore to have it is not in vaine.

Tusser also recommended that wormwood should be 'laid among stuffs and furs to keep away moths and insects'. The Greeks believed the plant was an antidote to hemlock poisoning, toadstools and the biting of the 'sea-dragon'. Wormwood is extremely bitter, but in the past it was used by brewers, before the advent of hops, because its leaves delayed the souring of ale. This same property made wormwood a principal ingredient in antiseptic preparations, although, to medieval medicine, the idea of antiseptics wasn't understood. They simply realised that herbs such as meadowsweet and wormwood helped ward off 'wound fever' – or sepsis, as we would call it. Wormwood was also recommended against the falling sickness (epilepsy) and for flatulence, as well as a good remedy for enfeebled digestion and debility.[16] Today, we know that the plant is full of quite powerful chemicals, including absinthol, absinthic acid and a bitter glucoside, absinthin. From this brief list, you've probably realised that wormwood is the key ingredient that flavours the potent drink absinthe.

On a lighter note, wormwood was also an ingredient in an old wives' love potion:

> On St. Luke's Day (18 October), take marigold flowers, a sprig of marjoram, thyme, and a little wormwood; dry them before a fire, rub them to powder; then sift it through a fine piece of lawn, and simmer it over a slow fire, adding a small quantity of virgin honey and vinegar. Anoint yourself with this when you go to bed, saying the following lines three times, and you will dream of your partner that is to be: 'St. Luke, St. Luke, be kind to me / In dreams let me my true-love see'.[17]

Nettles were considered a good treatment for 'thinness of the blood' and today can be bought in tablet form as the first-line therapy for anaemia. Comfrey leaves were commonly used as a poultice for muscular and/or skeletal injuries, its common name in folklore being 'knitbone'. The apothecary's rose was grown so the red petals could be used to make an effective antiseptic salve for cuts and deeper wounds. That gardener's foe, ground elder, was planted intentionally in medieval gardens because it can be infused as a tea or pounded into an ointment, both of which are excellent in the treatment of gout. As a drink, it flushes the kidneys thoroughly so is also good for general kidney problems. Every part of the plant can be used and is so effective in treating and even curing gout that it is used in modern medicine for the same purpose – perhaps not such a foe after all. It is clear that trial and error must have formed a very large part of the medical practice of the day but, over time, a detailed understanding of the actions of plant medicines developed.

In medieval times it was believed that smallpox occurred in young people because they had an excess of blood that flowed so fast it eventually boiled, bursting through the skin in red pustules. Therefore, the treatment consisted of a cooling diet of barley broth and removal of the excess humour by bloodletting, especially from the bridge of the nose to reduce the heat in the area of the brain. An interesting medical procedure, from tenth-century Japan to fourteenth-century England to nineteenth-century Denmark, was 'the red treatment' for this disease. It involved wrapping the patient in red cloth, draping the bedchamber with red hangings and red curtains drawn across the windows. The patient was encouraged to drink red-coloured fluids. John of Gaddesden (*c.* 1280–1349, one source gives the year of his death as 1361) was the royal physician to Edward II and treated the king's second son, John, Earl of Cornwall, when he suffered from smallpox, saying that he encouraged the patient to suck on a red pomegranate and gargle with red mulberry wine.[18] He wrote a treatise of medicine, the *Rosa Medicinae*, also referred to as *Rosa Anglica*, that became very popular in England. In it he notes what he did for the 'King's son', treating him by what he called the *scarletta rubra* method:

Then take a scarlet or other red cloth and wrap the smallpox patient up completely in it, as I did with the most noble King of England's son when this disease seized him, and I permitted only red things to be about his bed, by the which I cured him, without leaving a trace of the smallpox pustules on him.[19]

Originally, 'scarlet' wasn't a colour; it was a very expensive and fine woollen cloth. Because of its high quality, it was of course dyed with only the best, longest-lasting dyes and these were royal blue, royal purple and crimson, known as 'kermes' from the dried insects that produced it. Over time, the red dye became the most usual colour for scarlet cloth and, gradually, the name of the cloth came to mean the colour as well.

In 1562, aged twenty-nine, Queen Elizabeth I caught smallpox. At first her physicians thought she had a cold, but she developed a raging fever and the pustules began to appear. Like her royal forebear, she too was wrapped in red blankets. This may sound like a rather silly idea, that 'red' could cure the disease and leave the patient unscarred, but Elizabeth wasn't badly pockmarked, although the Lady Mary Dudley, a lady-in-waiting who attended the queen during her illness, was less fortunate. She caught the disease from the queen and was severely scarred, especially on her face. Did they fail to swathe her in red? Perhaps. In the last century, a Danish doctor, Neils Finson, writing in 1901 on the uses of ultraviolet light in medicine, noted,

[Smallpox patients placed] in rooms from which the [UV] rays ... are excluded by interposing red glass or thick red cloth, ... the vesicles [spots] as a rule do not enter upon the stage of suppuration and the patients get well with no scars at all, or at most with extremely slight scarring.[20]

Although Finsen won the Nobel Prize for showing how ultraviolet light could be used as a successful treatment for certain skin complaints, further studies of his red-light treatment for smallpox proved less convincing. However, clinical trials are ongoing into a red-light acne treatment with promising results so far,[21] so it is possible that John of Gaddesden and his fellow physicians were not so wide of the mark with their 'red treatment' for smallpox.

Other Useful Treatments – Antiseptics, Anaesthetics and Antibiotics

Today we take these things for granted and most likely assume that the first two were invented in the nineteenth century and that the third was a twentieth-century innovation. In name, that is probably the case – no medieval manuscript says 'for antiseptic purposes' or 'to make an anaesthetic' – but such things were known about, even if they weren't understood. The ancient Egyptians understood that mummifying bodies for the afterlife required the use of specific substances to prevent decay. They used pitch and turpentine, both of which were later used by surgeons, applied to amputated limb stumps. Although the word 'antiseptic' was first used by English physician Sir John Pringle (1707–82), Hippocrates had understood the concept, advising washing wounds with wine and vinegar and smearing them with oils, all of which have antiseptic properties. The ancient Persians had laws that required drinking water to be stored in copper vessels.[22] Copper acts as an antiseptic so the water stayed sweet and drinkable for much longer. It was recently realised that old Victorian brass banisters and handrails in public buildings are far more hygienic than those made of other, more modern materials, because brass has a high copper content. Here is an antiseptic ointment for treating inflamed wounds from the fifteenth century:

> For fester in a wound and dead flesh to destroy. Take new wax, verdigris, code [cobblers' wax], frankincense and pitch and tar, turpentine, sheep's tallow with grease and fry that

together in a pan; and when it is seethed together, cool it through a colander and put it in boxes.[23]

Every ingredient in this recipe either has antiseptic properties or is included to give a greasy ointment consistency that will seal the wound. (Verdigris is a blue-green chemical consisting mainly of copper hydroxide and copper carbonate that forms when brass, bronze and copper are weathered. As well as being a wonderful colour that was used in medieval painting, it is also an excellent antiseptic.)

Many people today believe anaesthetics are a modern invention and that all medieval surgery must, therefore, have caused the patient the most excruciating pain, but this isn't entirely true. We saw in a previous chapter a recipe for 'dwale' to put a patient to sleep before undergoing a surgical procedure. Here is another anaesthetic potion with instructions and dosage, which is unusual and shows how important it was in this case to give the patient just enough hemlock to make him sleep and no more, diluting it well in ale or wine:

To put a man to sleep that he may be treated or cut [operated upon]. Take the gall of a swine three spoonfuls and take the juice of hemlock-root three spoonfuls, of vinegar three spoonfuls and mingle all together and then put them in a vessel of glass to hold to the sick man that thou wilt treat or cut. And take thereof a spoonful and put it to a gallon of wine or ale. And if thou wilt make it strong, put two spoonfuls thereof and give him to drink and he shall sleep soon. Then mayest thou treat or cut him as thou wilt.[24]

Among the operations that were carried out successfully were procedures to remove cataracts from the eyes, nose polyps, haemorrhoids and harelip. This last was thought to happen to a baby if its mother had been unfortunate enough to see a hare during her pregnancy. Here are the Anglo-Saxon Bald's instructions for treating harelip:

> Mash mastic very small, add egg white, mingle as thou dost vermilion [i.e. mixing a pigment for illuminating a manuscript], cut with a knife the false lip edges, sew tight with silk, smear all over with the salve, ere the silk rot.[25]

Although the way antibiotics work has only been understood since the twentieth century, that doesn't mean they weren't used long before that. Sphagnum moss – used by flower arrangers today – has been a vital component in the surgeons' equipment bags for centuries. A skeleton from the Bronze Age, found in Scotland, had evidence of a large pad of sphagnum moss applied to a chest wound.[26] This bog moss, found in Scotland, Ireland and western England, is capable of soaking up fluids or discharge from a wound far better than cotton wool and deodorises it as well. These benefits would have been obvious, but what couldn't be known to the surgeons of history was that certain penicillin moulds live in the sphagnum moss, giving it antibiotic properties.

Something else unusual was used in treating wounds: spiders' webs or cobwebs. A ball of clean cobwebs would be used to pack an open wound and cover it, being able to stick to the skin because it is covered in natural glue and worked like sticking plaster. The webbing gradually dried and hardened, sealing and protecting the injury. As well as being incredibly strong and lightweight, when it had done its job it was easy to wash away with warm water. As an added benefit, spiders' webs have natural antiseptic and antifungal properties to combat infection. Finally, they also helped stop the bleeding and promoted the healing of the wound because they contain vitamin K, necessary in the process of clotting blood and repair. So long as the cobwebs were fresh and clean when they were applied, they wouldn't have caused any adverse reactions in the patient, being biologically neutral.[27] Though they had no knowledge of the reasons why cobwebs worked so well, trial and error had proved that they did so the medieval surgeon put them to good use.

Electuaries were medicinal syrups made with either honey or, for the wealthy, sugar. The importance of honey in medicine is recorded in some of the world's oldest medical literature. Since ancient times, it has been known for its wound-healing activity. An extra benefit the ancient healers wouldn't have understood, although they could have seen the results, was its antibacterial activity. Honey also keeps the wound from becoming stiff and too dry and its high viscosity (stickiness) helps to provide a protective barrier to prevent infection. It even gives the immune system a boost which helps wound repair too. The antimicrobial activity in most honeys is due to the presence of hydrogen peroxide, which inhibits the growth of bacteria and its high sugar content (high osmolarity), which draws the fluids out of any bacteria present, so they shrivel and die. This ability is bringing honey back into medical use today, not only as a wound dressing, but because of its antibiotic properties which act on bacteria in a number of ways, making it more difficult for the microbes to evolve a resistance to its effects.[28] Here are the instructions to a medieval apothecary for making electuaries for sale:

> Electuaries for divers evils. Take honey that is clarified and seethe it; and to know when it is seethed enough, take a drop thereof and let it fall in cold water: and if it be hard between thy fingers, then it is enough. And put therein powder of bay, a quarter of an ounce of ginger, half an ounce of long pepper and the same quantity of canell [cinnamon], and colour it with saunders [sandalwood, which was used as a red food colouring and smelled nice] and sell it forth.[29]

This electuary is described as especially suitable for treating 'rising and ache at the heart', which sounds like a love potion of some kind but was how they termed indigestion and heartburn in the fifteenth century.

With all these sensible, effective remedies being known and used by medieval practitioners, we have to admit that some treatments sound absurd, useless, revolting and, possibly in some cases, lethal, so let's look at some of those.

Outrageous Medicine and Treatments

Anglo-Saxon medicine frequently involved magic charms, spells and even daisy chains. These simple little flower garlands were put around a baby's neck to keep the fairies and mischievous sprites away. A childish tantrum could be explained as the influence of a bad fairy up to no good, so a necklace of 'day's eyes' kept the dark powers at bay. Other plants had similar uses, like sage and the bitter herb rue, and trees like the rowan warded off witches. Whether or not such precautions actually did any good, at least they did no harm, but some medicinal remedies, effective or not, definitely harmed members of the local animal community. A remedy for women who suffered from dysmenorrhoea (painful periods) required taking a cat, cutting off its head, removing its innards and laying the still warm body of the feline on the painful belly (from the *Fifteenth-century Leechbook*, recipe 238, p. 89). The warmth may have helped, but why not just sit with the live cat on your lap? The effect would be the same and the animal would still be available when needed next time, like a living hot-water bottle. Gout seems to have been an ailment that called for all manner of curious remedies:

> To cure gout. Boil a red-haired dog alive in oil until it falls apart. Then add worms, hog's marrow and herbs. Apply the mixture to the affected parts. Or take a frog when neither

sun nor moon is shining. Cut off its hind legs and wrap them in deer skin. Apply the right to the right and the left to the left foot of the gouty person and without doubt he will be healed.[30]

Gilbertus Anglicus recommended an ointment made from boiled puppy, cucumber, rue and juniper berries. John Mirfield (d. 1407) was a physician at St Bartholomew's Hospital, at Smithfield in London. He wrote a medical treatise, the *Breviarium Bartholomei*, an instruction book to be used at the hospital, dealing with health problems from head to toe. Among his general treatments, he included this gruesome medicinal bath:

Take blind puppies (i.e. too young to have their eyes open), gut them and cut off the feet, then boil in water and in this water let the patient bathe. Let him stay in the bath for four hours after he has eaten and while in the bath, he should keep his head covered and his chest swathed with the skin of a goat so he does not catch a sudden chill.[31]

Incidentally, Mirfield also includes the formula for a 'powder for that warlike or diabolic instrument that commonly is termed the gun' – gunpowder in other words.[32]

Baked owl was another remedy for gout (from the *Fifteenth-century Leechbook,* recipe 655, p. 207). Perhaps somewhat less barbaric than these recipes was a preparation of crushed ants. Dead puppies or dead mice as headache treatments, spiders for earache and cats for quinsy (severe tonsilitis) – all were recommended medieval treatments, but if they worked it was most likely down to the placebo effect. Here is another outrageous remedy (no. 40) for madness from Bald's *Leechbook*: for that one be moon-mad, take a mereswine's fel (a dolphin's skin), make it into a scourge (whip) and beat the man. He will soon be well. Amen.

We may think that such weird animal-based remedies are things of the distant past, but in fact similar strange possibilities from the animal kingdom are still being explored by researchers today.

Weird but Wonderful Treatments

Modern medicine now uses leeches and maggots have made a comeback for debriding (removing dead tissue) and cleaning wounds. In maggot debridement therapy, as it is called, clinically bred larvae of the green bottle blowfly are used to treat infected wounds in soft tissue and skin. The maggots are applied to the wound for two or three days, enclosed within special dressings to keep them from straying too far from the site being treated. Since these medicinal maggots cannot dissolve or feed on healthy tissue, their natural instinct is to crawl elsewhere as soon as the wounds are clean, or the larvae have eaten their fill.

Science has discovered that the maggots work in three ways: they debride (clean) the wound by dissolving dead and infected tissue with their digestive enzymes; they disinfect the wound (kill bacteria) by secreting antimicrobial molecules, by ingesting and killing microbes; and they stimulate the growth of new, healthy tissue.[33] They are proving especially successful in cleaning and healing leg ulcers associated with diabetes and in wounds caused by antibiotic-resistant bacteria, such as MRSA. In medieval times, the use of maggots probably happened by accident, rather than intent, but they do get mentioned, usually being called 'worms'.

In modern medical research, some very surprising creatures are providing chemical compounds for study. Exenatide is a synthetised drug, but was originally derived from a hormone found in the venomous saliva of the Gila monster, a large North American lizard. The drug is currently used as a successful treatment for type 2 diabetes.[34] Eristostatin, extracted from the venom of the Asian sand viper, is boosting patients' immune systems in the fight against malignant melanoma. Crotoxin, a protein extracted from rattlesnake venom, is being looked at as a possible future cancer treatment because it seems to trigger apoptosis in abnormal cells. Apoptosis is the self-destruct mechanism that deletes healthy cells at the end of their individual lifespan; a function that cancerous cells lack, enabling them to multiply out of control. King cobra toxin is providing an incredible analgesic (painkiller), hannalgesin, believed to be between twenty and two hundred times more effective than morphine. Clinical trials are ongoing.[35]

The origins of these new medicines are a reminder that we shouldn't dismiss out of hand some of the weird ingredients used in medieval remedies. It may be that some contain active compounds still to be discovered by modern researchers. After all, who would have rated lizard spit as a treatment for diabetics?

We cannot talk about animal-based remedies without mentioning dragon's blood. Dragon's blood isn't animal-related at all; it is a red resin from the tree *Dracaena draco*, which is native to the Canary Islands and Morocco. When the bark is damaged, the tree oozes a blood-red sap which hardens to protect the site of injury. Sold by medieval merchants as either lumps of dark-red resin or a bright-red powder, its cost was hugely increased by the incredible story told of its origins. According to these tales, trees were not involved at all. The resin was the solidified blood of dragons, slain in combat by their mortal enemies, elephants. Apparently the elephants were always victorious, which may explain why they are so much more common than dragons today.

Dragon's blood was used as a dye and a paint pigment as well as having medicinal properties. The Greek botanist-physician Dioscorides described its uses in his herbal, *De Materia Medica*, advising it for respiratory and gastrointestinal problems, particularly for diarrhoea. Trotula of Salerno – who may or may not have been a female lecturer in medicine at the University of Salerno in the twelfth century – recommended it in a long list of ingredients to make a remedy for treating women who suffer menorrhagia (heavy bleeding during their periods): 'After eating or during meals, let there be given to them to drink ... a powder of coral and gum arabic, pomegranate, myrtleberry seed and purslane ... great plantain, knotgrass, dragon's blood, burnt elephant bones and quince seed.'[36]

By 1402, dragon's blood was known to come from a plant, but it was still used in medicine as a cure-all. It was applied to wounds as a coagulant, to stop the bleeding, for reducing fevers, curing diarrhoea and dysentery. It was taken by mouth for mouth ulcers, sore throats, intestinal and stomach disorders, as well as for chest problems. It was also applied to the skin as an eczema treatment. But did this exotic substance have any beneficial effects? The answer is yes, it probably did. Today, alternative medicine uses dragon's blood as an antiseptic wash for wounds and internally for chest pains, menstrual problems and post-partum bleeding after childbirth. More orthodox medical research has found that dragon's blood has not only antibiotic properties, but one of its components, taspine, has antiviral and wound-healing effects.[37] Animal and laboratory tests have shown some promise for the use of dragon's blood in modern medicine but, to date, there are no human clinical studies verifying these effects.

These days, dragon's blood resin is still imported – at one time it was used to varnish Stradivarius violins – but *Dracaena draco* is just one source. The resin can also be obtained from *Dracaena cinnabari*, which is native to the island of Socotra in the Indian Ocean, and this may well have been another source available to Islamic medicine and to Europe via the Incense Road. Most supplies now come from various species of *Daemonorops*, native to Malaysia and Indonesia.

One other unlikely sounding animal-based remedy was snail or slug slime. The mucus excretion of a live snail was recommended by medieval apothecaries as an immediate treatment for burns and scalds, minor injuries, itchy skin and also for dissolving warts. In the case of burns and scalds, it was supposed to reduce blistering and ease the pain. Recent research has shown that snail slime contains antioxidants, antiseptic, anaesthetic, anti-irritant, anti-inflammatory, antibiotic and antiviral properties, as well as collagen and elastin, vital for skin repair. As with leech saliva, these chemical compounds are all for the creature's benefit. Imagine a snail or slug sliding over gritty ground or rough plant material; it must suffer minor scratches and abrasions that could easily cause discomfort or become infected. Modern science now utilises snail slime, under the heading 'Snail Gel', as skin preparations and for treating minor injuries, such as cuts, burns and scalds. It is also being trialled as a wart remover. It seems that medieval medicine got this one right.[38]

Mandrake

This strange plant, mentioned in the Old Testament of the Bible, may be familiar to *Harry Potter* fans as a dangerous magical thing, able to drive to madness anyone who hears it scream as it is uprooted. In the book of Genesis[39] Leah, who thought she was past childbearing, conceives by using mandrake to make her fertile again, so medieval people would have been familiar with the plant. However, legends grew up around mandrake with its strange taproot in the branching shape of something almost human-looking. Although the Bible story says simply that Reuben found the plants growing in the wheatfield and 'brought them unto his mother Leah', presumably without any unforeseen consequences for him, myths were told about the mandrake, that when pulled from the ground it shrieked terribly, causing any living creature within earshot to go insane and die. To guard against this, herb gatherers would tie a dog to the plant and make a quick exit from the scene. When the dog pulled on the string in an attempt to follow, eventually its struggles would uproot the plant with the terminal outcome for the unfortunate animal. Did people really believe this story, even when the dogs survived their task? More likely it was a cautionary tale because the plant is related to belladonna (deadly nightshade) and similarly toxic.

Nevertheless, it was used in medieval medicine. Seen as a universal cure and an infallible charm against evil, mandrake has analgesic and sleep-inducing properties. In Roman times, it was sometimes given as an act of mercy, by means of a wine-soaked sponge, to those undergoing execution by crucifixion.[40] Trotula of Salerno advised using mandrake to treat various afflictions of the womb, along with belladonna and henbane – a deadly trio of ingredients if not used sparingly and with the greatest care.[41] According to Trotula, mandrake was also a vital ingredient in two important remedies. The first, populeon, was an ointment based on ground poplar buds and pork fat. It was ideal for treating acute fever or insomnia and should be rubbed into the patient's abdomen. The recipe included mandrake leaves – no need to uproot the plant in this case – henbane, lettuce (a soporific), black nightshade and violets.[42] The second, potio Sancti Pauli, was a potion to be drunk by the patient and had, supposedly, been invented by St Paul. It was a treatment for epilepsy, catalepsy and stomach problems. The extensive list of components included licorice, sage, willow, roses, three kinds of pepper, fennel, cinnamon, ginger, cloves, cormorant blood, mandrake and dragon's blood.[43]

Apart from these treatments in Trotula's writings, for all its fame I have found the mandrake plant to be quite elusive and not only in medieval medicine. On two occasions, visits to the Chelsea Physic Garden in London to photograph the growing plants resulted in disappointment. The first visit in early September 2013 proved to be too late in the season because mandrake dies back completely – not so much as a withered leaf remains above the ground. All that was visible was the label, 'Mandrake or Mandragora officinalis', to show where it grew. Not wanting to miss it a second time, a return visit to the garden in May 2014 was equally unrewarding. After the wettest winter on record with mild temperatures, slugs and snails were having a wonderful year. Not so their favourite plant foods, including mandrake. Enquiries revealed one well-chewed mandrake shoot, about as tall as my finger, struggling in the rockery garden. Therefore, this book is lacking a photograph of this legendary plant. The snails probably benefitted from its supposed aphrodisiac qualities – they certainly weren't killed off by its toxicity.

Treacle for the Rich

For the most serious diseases, prevention was always better than cure, but some concoctions were reckoned to do both. The following was written by an anonymous chronicler, describing how the lives of the people of Winchester were saved when plague came to the city in 1471:

> The most sovereyn medycyn for the pestilence concludyd be doctures of fesycke both beyonde the se and yn Ynglond also a bowte the kyng yn late days yn the reyngne of Kyng Edward the iiijth the xth yere [1471].Take ij sponefuls of water and j sponeful of vinygar and treacle the size of a bean and mix alle this to gedyr and drynke hit fasting once a week or twice yn a month and yf yow are not infected hit will preserve yow and yf yow are infected hit will save yowr lyfe with regular habyts. This is proved and has saved 300 or 400 lyfes of men, women and children yn the city of Winchester yn the yere of the kyng abovesaid.

This recipe sounds so cheap and easy. If it prevented and cured plague why should anyone die of that dreaded disease? Water, vinegar and treacle sound simple enough. The trouble was this 'treacle' wasn't any old treacle. It was 'theriac'. According to legend, the history of theriac begins with King Mithridates VI, King of Pantus (now in Turkey) in the second century BC, who had a great fear of being assassinated by poison.[44] To be certain of having the correct antidote, if anyone ever did succeed in poisoning him, he experimented with every known poison and all possible antidotes on his prisoners. His numerous toxicity experiments eventually led him to declare that he had discovered an antidote for every venomous reptile and poisonous substance. He then mixed all the effective antidotes into a single one, which he called 'mithridate', naming this incredible cure-all after himself. Mithridate contained opium, myrrh, saffron, ginger, cinnamon and castor oil, along with some forty other ingredients.

When the Romans defeated Mithridates, his medical notes fell into their hands and Roman *medici* began to use them. Emperor Nero's physician, Andromachus, improved upon mithridate by bringing the total number of ingredients to sixty-four, including viper's flesh, a mashed decoction of which, first roasted then well aged, proved the most constant ingredient. Apparently, the Roman emperor Marcus Aurelius took it on a regular basis on the advice of his physician, Galen. After all, he was wealthy and could afford all those expensive ingredients.

In the medieval period, the traditional name became corrupted and shortened to 'theriac' and this, the most expensive of all medicaments, now with more than a hundred ingredients, was called Venice or Genoa treacle by the English, depending on which Italian city state they imported it from. Along with two other Officinal Capitals, or magic bullets as we would call them – Philonium, which contained saffron, pyrethrum, pepper and honey; and Dioscordium, which contained ginger, cinnamon, cassia, opium, gentian and honey among other things[45] – theriac was still believed to cure everything from snake bite to jaundice, leprosy to intestinal wounds. It simply kept 'the entire body incorrupt'.[46] However, even if you could afford this 'sovereign medicine' or 'magic bullet' the secret of success lay in those two words 'regular habits'. What were one man's perfect regular habits could be another man's destruction, depending on his humoral complexion, so the outcome was still in doubt, even for the rich. As for the common folk, there was no chance of them getting hold of even that 'bean-sized' amount of treacle, enough for a single dose and, when it came to their 'regular habits', of course they were deplorably irregular in every way. Especially irregular in their habits were women – ever unpredictable – so in the next chapter we will turn our attention to them, in their roles as both carers and patients.

7

WHEN THE DOCTOR – OR
THE PATIENT – IS A WOMAN

When a woman is making love with a man, a sense of heat
   in her brain,
which brings with it sensual delight, communicates the taste
   of that
delight during the act and summons forth the emission of
   the man's seed.

Hildegard of Bingen (1098–1179)

You may be surprised to learn that the woman who wrote this
description of a female orgasm was a nun! Hildegard of Bingen
wrote poetry, drama and music, about the politics of her day,
made various prophesies and, most relevant for us, wrote treatises
about herbs and medicine. She was quite an extraordinary woman,
who exerted a tremendous influence – both temporal and spiritual
– on her time. Hildegard was born in 1098 in Bockelheim, in the
diocese of Mainz in Germany. Her father, Hildebert, was a knight
in the service of Meginhard, the Count of Spanheim. At the age of
six, little Hildegard began to have religious visions which would
continue for the rest of her life. Two years later, she was given into
the care of Jutta, sister of Count Meginhard. Jutta and her foster

daughter lived in a small cottage beside the church in the abbey founded by St Disibode at Disibodenberg. Although she wasn't a particularly healthy child, Hildegard nevertheless studied hard under Jutta's tutelage, learning to read, write and sing in Latin.

At the age of fifteen, she took her vows and became a nun. Jutta, who by this time had attracted enough followers to form a community, set up a convent, following the Rule of St Benedict, with herself as the abbess. When Jutta died in 1136, Hildegard, at the age of thirty-eight, became the new abbess.

As her visions continued, she explained them to her confessor, a monk named Godfrey. Godfrey spoke to his abbot who brought them to the attention of the Archbishop of Mainz. He and his theologians examined her visions, ruled that they were divinely inspired and that Hildegard should record them in writing. In the year 1141, she began her principal work, *Scivias*, which means 'May You Know the Way', completing it in 1151. Even Pope Eugenius III got to hear about Hildegard. Because of her new-found fame, the community at Disibodenberg soon outgrew its little convent so it was moved to Rupertsberg near Bingen. Here, Hildegard oversaw the building of a large convent which could easily accommodate the growing number of women attracted to her community. She remained at Bingen – except during her extensive travels in western Europe – did most of her writing there and continued as abbess until her death on 17 September 1179, aged eighty-one. She was buried in her convent church, where her relics remained until 1632 when the convent was destroyed by the invading Swedish army and her relics moved to Eibingen.

A woman of incredible energy with a uniquely independent mind, Hildegard wrote voluminously. *Scivias* was only the first of her three mystical works based on her visions, but is full of useful ideas. In *Scivias*, she developed her views on the universe and, more important for medicine, the structure of humans, the processes of birth and death and the nature of the soul and its relationship with the body and to God. The last of her twenty-six visions in this first book is the earliest morality play yet to be discovered.

Hildegard's third work – *The Book of the Divine Works of a Simple Man* – was written between 1163 and 1173 and is all about the unity of creation. In it she sets her theological beliefs alongside her knowledge of the elements of the universe and the structures within the human body. At the time, this book was the ultimate in scientific writing and it was here that her ideas on medicine and natural science were set out and where she elaborated on the medical and cosmic interrelationship of humanity and the world in great detail. Between 1151 and 1158, she wrote her medical work *Of the Simplicities of Various Natural Creatures*. The original of this work hasn't been discovered but both the *Book of Simple Medicine* and the *Book of Compound Medicine – Causes and Cures* are wonderfully preserved in a thirteenth-century manuscript discovered in the Royal Library in Copenhagen in 1859.

The work we are mainly interested in here is Hildegard's *Physica*, particularly the section on 'Plants'. There are eight other sections, on 'Elements, Trees, Stones, Fish, Birds, Animals, Reptiles and Metals'. The first section contains 230 chapters on the medicinal uses of plants and this comprehensiveness suggests that she took particular interest in healing plants and was most probably practising medicine herself. Yet it is difficult to decide whether she was wholly relying on her own experience, traditional folklore or written authorities. If she did use earlier authorities, though, they weren't the usual Pliny and Dioscorides for there is virtually no overlap of information. On the other hand, the plants she writes of and used were generally those that could be collected from the woods and fields around or grown in the convent garden, although more exotic ingredients for her medications, like ginger, pepper, incense and sugar, must have been purchased.

Hildegard made little attempt to describe the plants for purposes of identification and she assumed, rather than spelled out, the medical and physiological theories behind their uses. She did, however, follow the traditional view that created things consisted of mixtures of the four elements – hot, cold, wet and dry – in which one or two qualities predominated. She combined these elements with the theological idea, ultimately taken from the biblical book of Genesis, according to which everything on earth was put there by God for the use of mankind. Since the balance of the elements and their corresponding humours determined good or bad health in people, it was essential to know the elemental qualities of plants before using them in an effort to restore the humoral balance of a sick person. Therefore, the most important information Hildegard gave about the plants was whether they were hot or cold – the opposing qualities that were the most significant for medical purposes. She then usually indicated what purposes each plant served; sometimes this followed fairly obviously from its qualities, at other times the connection was more tenuous. Here are Hildegard's ideas on the uses of a couple of well-known plants:

Rose is cold and this same coldness has a useful temperament in it. At daybreak or in the morning, take a rose leaf and place it over your eye; this draws out the humour and makes it clear. But let whoever has a weeping ulcer on his or her body, place a rose leaf over it and draw out the pus. But rose also strengthens any potion or ointment or any other medication when it is added to it. And these are so much better even if only a little rose has been added to them. This is from the good strength of the rose, as previously mentioned.

Sage is warm and dry of nature. It grows more from the warmth of the sun than from the humidity of the earth. It is useful against sick humours since it is dry. Take sage and pulverise it. Eat this powder with bread and it diminishes the overabundance of bad humours in you … But let whoever is worn out by stiffness cook sage in water and drink it ... and it checks the stiffness. For if it is given with wine, the wine makes the stiffening humours pass by in some way.

As you can see, Hildegard knew her stuff when it came to using medicinal plants, at least by the reckoning of the day, but let's return to that epigraph at the top of this chapter, concerning women and sex. We will have to leave aside the fact that a woman – indeed, one who spent all but the first six years of her life as a nun in a state of chastity – seemed to know all about the female orgasm, and look at why she thought it was a subject that ought to be included in a book on medicine. Medieval people believed that, in order for a woman to conceive a child, it wasn't only necessary for the man to reach orgasm and ejaculate, but for the woman to also achieve orgasm in order to release her 'contribution' to the baby's make-up. Exactly what form the woman's 'contribution' took was still a mystery, but they were certain it was vital. In marriage, this was a definite bonus for the wife; if he wanted heirs, the husband had to ensure that his partner enjoyed the lovemaking as much as he did. However, if a woman was unfortunate enough to be raped and became pregnant as a result, then it couldn't have been rape because she must have been a willing participant, else she wouldn't have conceived.

Incredibly, quite recently, a US politician declared that he wouldn't support the issue of abortion for rape victims for precisely this reason. William Todd Akin, a former US Representative in Congress, serving from 2001 to 2013, ended his career after he lost an election he had seemed about to win. His downfall happened when he said that women who are victims of what he called 'legitimate rape' rarely get pregnant. Akin eventually apologised for the remark, but in a book that he published in July 2014, he said he regretted having made the apology and defended his original comments.[1]

Trotula – The Mystery of Another Woman in Medicine

A little after Hildegard's time, in the twelfth century, there may – or may not – have been a woman known to history as Trotula of Salerno. Some historians believe she was a lecturer at the medical faculty in the University of Salerno in Italy, a little way down the coast from Naples, and that she wrote extensively on women's medical conditions and requirements and even about cosmetics. But others think that 'Trotula' must have been a *nom de plume* used by male physicians who preferred to remain anonymous when writing about such a controversial subject, one that they usually avoided otherwise. The reason given is that the text was too good to have been written by a mere woman. Conversely, yet another scholar writes that the text was so poor that the male author was ashamed of it, so he put a woman's name on it. The subject of authorship is still open to debate.

Today there are supporters in both camps, but in medieval times we find references to the works of 'Dame Trot' and her books, *On the Conditions of Women, On Treatments for Women,* and *On Women's Cosmetics*, dotted about in various medical treatises, even in England, though they aren't always attributed to her. Nevertheless, modern scholars understand that, in medieval times, plagiarism was not only frequent but demanded, and many unacknowledged recipes and treatments have been traced back to the writings of Trotula. At least we know someone named Trotula was listed on the register of citizens of Salerno[2] around the appropriate dates, but this could be a coincidence.

Trotula wrote extensively about menstruation, conception, pregnancy and birth. Some of her advice sounds rather odd today, such as her test to discover whether the husband or wife is at fault if she fails to conceive. This required two identical pots of wheat bran. The husband's urine was used to soak the bran in one pot and the wife's to soak the other. Whichever went rotten first, that spouse was the partner at fault.[3] This was a radical idea of Trotula's – that the husband might be to blame if the woman didn't become pregnant. She also thought it was possible to choose whether the woman would conceive a boy child or a girl, so the instructions went on:

> If she wishes to conceive a male, let her husband take the womb and vagina of a hare and let him dry them, and let him mix the powder with wine and drink it. Similarly, let the woman do the same thing with the testicles of a hare and at the end of her period let her lie with her husband and then she will conceive a male.

This most probably worked in about 50 per cent of cases.

Galen had explained how, in the male body, some blood was transformed into semen, but in women, because their bodies had less heat, they weren't so efficient at converting blood and so could produce only a little inferior semen. The blood 'left over' in women was used to nourish the growing foetus and, later, after the child was born, the excess was transformed into milk. If a woman didn't bear a child, the extra blood had to be disposed of; that was why women menstruated. Following these assumptions, some medieval anatomical drawings show veins or ducts to transfer the blood from the womb to the breasts to supply milk, and another vein through which menstrual blood supposedly flowed away. However, despite all these female 'failings', even the ancients had to acknowledge that only women's bodies were capable of producing children, but how did this process work?

Soranus, a Greek doctor in Rome in the first century AD, believed that a woman's womb was hotter and drier on the right side and wetter and colder on the left; therefore a child conceived on the right was male and, on the left, female. In the sixteenth century, Henry VIII could still blame his first two wives for failing to produce living male children because their wombs were too wet and cold throughout and, therefore, could only give birth to healthy girls.

Not surprisingly, the Church got involved in such matters as sex between a husband and wife. Firstly, the act was banned throughout the forty days of Lent, during Advent, the eve of many feast days and on Sundays or any weekday before attending Mass. Secondly, sex was for no other purpose than the creation of children, so it was not allowed if the woman was already pregnant or if she was past the menopause. Definitely forbidden was intercourse during a woman's 'unclean' time of her period and, if she should conceive at such a time – which was thought to be quite possible – she would bear the devil's child, made recognisable to all by its red hair. Little wonder then that the population of medieval Europe had barely made good its losses from the plague by the seventeenth century.

Trotula's advice for treating a woman, once she had succeeded in becoming pregnant, was that great care had to be taken 'to name nothing in her hearing which she may not have'.[4] The reason given was that she would set her mind on it and, if she didn't get it, her desire for it would cause a miscarriage. If she fancied strange things to eat, such as 'clay, chalk or coals', she should be given beans cooked with sugar to suppress the craving. If she suffered swollen ankles, they should be massaged with rose oil and vinegar. As the time of delivery approached, she should bathe frequently, rub her belly with olive oil or oil of violets and eat light and easily digestible meals. Trotula made these recommendations as means of relieving the pain of childbirth as far as possible. This idea directly contradicted the teaching of the Church that women were meant to endure the pain because of Eve's sinful behaviour in the Garden of Eden.[5]

A medical treatise written in French in 1256 for Beatrice of Savoy, Countess of Provence, by Aldobrandino of Siena is fascinating but only applicable to wealthy women, his advice being to refrain from work and from beating the servants – impossible

for poorer women. Aldobrandino thought the most risky times for
the pregnant woman were early on, during the first three months,
and as her time of confinement approached. He gave detailed
dietary instructions: to eat little and often, having white meats like
chicken, partridge, blackbird, kid and mutton, and drinking wine
with water. Pears, pomegranates and apples were recommended to
stimulate the appetite. Salty food was to be avoided or the baby
might be born without hair and fingernails. Electuaries (tonics in
the form of a conserve, usually made with honey) should be taken
to strengthen the body, although only the rich could have afforded
them, the recipes including ground pearls, ginger, cinnamon bark,
nutmeg and pepper. Mood and attitude were also important,
especially at the beginning and end of pregnancy, a joyful and
contented outlook was to be cultivated, while anger, fear and
trauma had to be banished from the mind. It was also inadvisable
to bathe too frequently, although washing generally was all right
and clothing should be clean and fresh, nor was the woman to stay
too long in the sun.

While in labour, if matters weren't progressing, Trotula
recommended the woman should take a bath in water in which
mallow, fenugreek, linseed and barley had been cooked and
her belly and vagina massaged with oil of roses or violets. She
suggested sneezing, brought on by inhaling frankincense powder,
might help force the baby out. Meanwhile, she should be walking
about at a slow pace.[6] If the baby was still reluctant to come out,
it could be persuaded by burning aromatic herbs and spices, for
instance mint and oregano, ambergris and aloewood, and wafting
the scented smoke into the vagina to tempt the child forth.[7] Trotula
explained exactly the mysteries of how the foetus developed in the
womb, according to medieval medical knowledge:

In the first month there is purgation of the blood. In the
second month there is expression of the blood and the body

[of the foetus]. In the third month it produces nails and hair. In the fourth month it begins to move and for that reason the woman is nauseated. In the fifth month the foetus takes on the likeness of its father or its mother. In the sixth month the nerves are constituted. In the seventh month the foetus solidifies its bones and nerves. In the eighth month Nature moves and the infant is made complete in the blessing of all its parts. In the ninth month it proceeds from the darkness into the light.[8]

Despite the inaccuracies in this description of events, I find it surprisingly lacking in religious connotations. There is no mention of any godly involvement in the creation and development of the foetus, but rather 'Nature' with a capital letter.

Once the child arrived, Trotula had lengthy instructions for its immediate care and on choosing a suitable wet nurse, swaddling and weaning. The first task of the midwife was to press back the ears of the newborn, so they didn't stick out and in order that (oddly) milk wouldn't get into the ear when it suckled. Then the umbilical cord had to be tied and cut at a three-finger distance from the belly. In the case of a boy child this was especially important because 'according to the retention of the umbilical cord the male member will be greater or smaller'. Any mucous secretions had to be wiped away and washed from around its nose and mouth with warm water, then its mouth and tongue anointed with honey 'so that it might talk the sooner'. The baby should be bathed and massaged daily after breast-feeding and its facial features straightened. Then it should be bandaged in linen to keep its limbs restrained, although Trotula recommended that it should sometimes be allowed to sleep without being confined in this swaddling. The newborn's eyes were to be shielded from strong light, but as it grew 'there should be different kinds of pictures, cloths of diverse colours and beads put in front of the child'; it should be sung to and talked to 'using neither rough nor harsh words' – instructions that sound quite modern. It would be nursed, bathed and changed every three hours and rubbed with rose oil.

Poorer women always breastfed their babies – the milk was free and not to be wasted – but Thomas of Chobham, writing in the early thirteenth century, was scathing about wealthy women who refused to breastfeed; he regarded this as a form of infanticide and described such negligent mothers as 'more cruel than beasts'. Yet wet nursing was widespread among the better-off in medieval Europe, partly because of the urgent need for more heirs. It was usual to breastfeed a child for at least two years and because they believed that breastfeeding prevented another pregnancy, the aristocracy didn't want such long interludes between their children's births – life was too short and unpredictable and confirming the inheritance of the family titles and estates was paramount. Trotula recommended a young and clean wet nurse, with a pink-and-white complexion, well built and with full breasts, who had given birth not too long before.

Trotula gives detailed instructions for the nurse's diet and, above all, she was not to eat garlic. Aldobrandino was also concerned over the nurse's character and urged that she should be cheerful, good-tempered, and shouldn't terrify the child. He also thought it important that the nurse's own child should have been a boy. This was because they thought the milk was different, according to whether the baby was a boy or girl; 'boy's' milk was somehow 'stronger'. If boy's milk was given to a girl child, she would grow to be rather a tomboy, so that was acceptable. The other way around – giving girl's milk to a boy child – would produce an effeminate, weakly male, which was not acceptable at all. Human breast milk, with these important characteristics, often appears as an ingredient in medical remedies. The child could be weaned from age two onwards on a pap of bread, honey and milk, to which Aldobrandino said 'a little wine might be added', the nurse softening the bread by chewing it herself.

During teething, the child's painful gums were to be soothed with a mixture of butter, goose grease and barley water. When weaning began, the child was to be given 'lozenges made from sugar and milk in the amount of an acorn … so it could hold them in its hand and play with them and suck on them'. Then the breast meat of hens, pheasants and partridges was the best food as breast milk was 'drawn away day by day'.

Having given birth to a healthy child, suppose the woman didn't want to get pregnant again for a while? In this case, Trotula's methods of birth control sound weird, harping back to the days of magic and sorcery:

> If a woman does not wish to conceive, let her carry against her nude flesh the womb of a goat which has never had offspring. Or there is found a certain stone called 'jet', which if it is held by the woman or even tasted prohibits conception. In another fashion, take a male weasel and let its testicles be removed and let it be released alive. Let the woman carry these testicles in her bosom and let her tie them in goose skin or in another skin and she will not conceive.[9]

Perhaps the goat's womb and weasel's testicles wrapped in goose skin were successful because, after a few days, they smelled so bad that both partners were put right off sex. As for the jet, which is only found at Whitby in Yorkshire, it is interesting to learn that this stone was known to Trotula in Italy, but as a method of birth control I cannot think that carrying it or licking it would have any effect. So the next problem might be an unwanted pregnancy. As we saw in chapter 6, the Hippocratic oath stated that a physician would not 'give a woman means to procure an abortion'. Even if he had not taken the oath, the Roman Catholic Church forbade abortion, as it still does today – and birth control, come to that. Just as in our time, there were always going to be women who, finding themselves 'with child', would do anything to escape the inevitable outcome, even at grave risk to their own lives. So medical practitioners were pragmatic; if the women were determined, it was better to do it as safely as possible by the standards of the day. For this reason, it isn't unusual to find in medieval medical texts remedies to 'restore the menses', i.e. to bring on a woman's periods. Without stating the obvious and offending holy Church, these were abortifacients – to abort the foetus from the womb. This is one of Trotula's remedies:

An excellent powder for provoking the menses: take some yellow flag [iris], hemlock, castoreum, mugwort, sea wormwood, myrrh, common centaury and sage. Let a powder be made and let her be given to drink one dram of this with water in which savin and myrrh are cooked and let her drink this in the bath.[10]

Castoreum comes from the scent glands of a beaver and savin is an extract of the poisonous tips of the leaves of *Juniper sabina*, in the past used as an anthelminthis – to get rid of intestinal worms – and known to be an abortifacient. As for drinking the dose while in the bath, that is reminiscent of the 'gin and a hot bath' old wives' method of abortion. With the addition of hemlock, if the woman survived the ordeal, most probably the pregnancy wouldn't and the remedy would be reckoned a success.

Unfortunately, numerous and frequent pregnancies, often from the age of twelve or so, made childbearing a great hazard for medieval women. Brewer explains that they were more than likely to suffer from anaemia and queens were no exception. He believes it is more than likely that Elizabeth of York – wife of Henry VII and mother of Henry VIII – died after giving birth to her seventh child because of anaemia, alongside the possibilities of postpartum infection and complications. Brewer believes that for menstruating and pregnant women, the medieval diet was severely lacking in iron. He claims that the women ate far less meat than the men, their diet consisting of mainly grain, vegetables and honey and the resulting deficiency of iron would mean that pregnancy and childbirth put an immense strain on both mother and baby.[11] Their resistance to infection would have been low and their strength taxed to the limits by the effort of birthing.

Brewer may be correct in his assumption that medieval women were prone to anaemia, but his assertion that their diet was to blame is difficult to substantiate. I have found no contemporary evidence that women ate less meat than men, at least in cases where it was plentiful. In poor families where meat was eaten rarely, it would quite likely have been the men who got the biggest portion and the women who went without, but in the royal and noble households meat would have been available to both sexes, Church regulations on days of fasting permitting. Elizabeth of York is unlikely to have been denied meat. As for a diet high in grain, vegetables and honey, the leafy vegetables would generally have had a reasonably good iron content.

We cannot leave Trotula without looking at some of her cosmetic treatments: waxing for hair removal, hair dyes, hair perfumes, conditioners and volumisers and even suntan lotion.[12] Waxing treatments seem to have been intended to remove unwanted facial hair, rather than underarms, legs or more intimate places. The wax was a mixture of Greek pitch (pine resin) and beeswax melted together with a few drops of galbanum (an aromatic gum resin from certain umbelliferous Persian plant species) and cooked over the fire 'for a long time, stirring with a spatula'. Mastic, frankincense and gum arabic were then added and the mixture left to cool. When it was lukewarm, it was applied to the face and left for an hour. When cold, it was removed, leaving the face beautiful, hairless and blemish free. To dye the hair black, recipes containing oak apples or walnut juice were listed and both would have worked. Incidentally, oak apples were also used to make medieval ink. If the woman preferred to go blonde, cabbage stalks and roots were to be pulverised together with shavings of boxwood or ivory, which made a golden-yellow powder to cleanse and colour the hair. As an alternative, the heartwood of a boxtree, broom flowers, crocus and egg yolks could be boiled in water and the surface scum used to anoint the hair and make it golden. Not only should a woman's hair look good, it should smell good too and Trotula advised musk and clove powder to be combed through the hair as the perfume of choice, 'but take care that it not be seen by anyone'.

An ointment to prevent sunburn was made from cooked lily-root, mastic powder, frankincense, camphor, white lead and pork grease, pounded to a powder and dissolved in rosewater. White lead was used by women from Roman times at least until the seventeenth century as a sort of foundation powder, despite the fact that it was known to be lethal – the ultimate price paid for being fashionable. The root of both red and white bryony mixed in honey could be used to redden the cheeks, perhaps at the risk of attracting wasps. Brazilwood in powdered alum created a lip dye, 'a most beautiful colour, combining red and white' – pink, presumably. To set off her new look, a woman was advised to chew fennel, lovage or parsley leaves, to give off a good smell, clean the gums and make the teeth very white.

Women as Medicinal Practitioners

If Trotula existed and was a university-qualified physician, she was virtually unique in medieval medicine. One other that we know of, once again in Italy, was Dorotea Bocchi.[13] She was the Professor of Medicine and Philosophy at the University of Bologna for more than forty years, from 1390 to 1436, having succeeded her father in the post. In medieval times and into the eighteenth century, Italy was far more liberal in such matters as the education of women. England lagged far behind, sadly. In this country, there were one or two references to female physicians, but they were labelled as charlatans and deceivers and, however knowledgeable they may have been, since the universities of Europe only admitted men, they ✓ couldn't have completed their studies in the traditional way.

In sixteenth-century Norwich, the Guild of Physicians and Barber-Surgeons complained about 'sundry women who were practising physic and surgery who were regarded as quacks'. At St Bartholomew's Hospital in Smithfield, London, and St Thomas's in Southwark, in 1562, Master Gale noted that the poor state of at least 300 patients at those hospitals was caused because they were being treated 'by witches, by women and by counterfeit rascals; three score women that occupieth the arte of physicke and chirurgery'[14]. But at least matters hadn't yet gone so far as they did in Salisbury in 1614, when the Company of Barber-Surgeons of the town specifically banned 'divers women and others within this city, altogether unskilful in the art of chirurgery who oftentimes take cures on them, to the great danger of the patient ... that no such woman or any other shall take or meddle with any cure of chirurgery'.[15]

However, in the medieval period, women were able to qualify as surgeons perfectly legitimately by working as apprentices, serving under other surgeons. Usually, the master was a relative of the woman – her father, uncle or elder brother, etc. The City of London regulations demanded that all apprentices signed an indenture to study under a master-surgeon for at least seven years to complete the course, learning the practical skills. Surgery was a craft, not an art like that of a physician. Because it didn't involve going to university and, therefore, require enrolment in holy orders, girls could serve an apprenticeship to practise surgery. The records suggest that there were never very many female surgeons, but a woman named only as 'Katherine' is listed as a surgeon in London in 1250. Apparently, her father and brothers were all surgeons too, so it seems she had followed in the family tradition. In 1389, London master surgeons were required to take an oath to keep 'faithful oversight of all others, both men and women, occupied in the art of surgery'. The annals of the Barber-Surgeons of London record, 'From the earliest times the custom has prevailed to admit women to the freedom [of the company of Barber-Surgeons] mostly by apprenticeship but also by patrimony, and these freewomen bound their apprentices, both boys and girls at the Hall [Guildhall].'[16]

Unfortunately, we know the names of hardly any women involved in this 'custom' from the fourteenth or fifteenth centuries in England and often they are only mentioned in passing with a derogatory comment. For example, in the late fourteenth century, the London surgeon, John of Arderne, wrote of a priest who had had a lump on his right breast for two years and consulted 'a lady' who instructed him to lay a plaster on it (to draw it out) and to drink 'the drynke of Antioche'. Then the priest consulted 'a wise surgeon' – meaning John of Arderne himself – who advised him not to use corrosive plasters. Another of Arderne's patients had also been consulting 'a lady' for six months and the drink of Antioch and 'other pillules' was all she could recommend.

Despite John of Arderne's reservations about women in medicine, his untitled medical treatise, which he wrote sometime after 1425, contains illustrations of a woman carrying out 'cupping' procedures on both male and female patients. Arderne's treatise is now in the British Library, catalogued as 'Sloane MS 6'. Folio 177r shows a fashionably gowned woman, wearing the latest in headdress design, cupping a naked man at various points all over his body. Folio 177v shows the same woman cupping a seated naked female patient beneath her breasts and on her abdomen. Historians have speculated that the well-dressed woman might be Arderne's wife, although nothing is mentioned in the treatise, so she remains anonymous.

In 1421, a group of London physicians petitioned the Privy Council in an effort to change the law so that 'no woman use the practice of Physick', but the council never obliged. One of very few positive references to a woman in medicine is found in the will of the wealthy London barber-surgeon Nicholas Bradmore, drawn up in 1417. Bradmore bequeaths a red belt with a silver buckle and 6*s* 8*d* to his apprentice Agnes Wodekok, whom he seems to remember with fondness.[17]

Midwives

There was one branch of medieval medicine, though, where women ruled: midwifery. Like those training for surgery, a girl would do an apprenticeship, working under an older, experienced midwife, and from her she would learn all she needed to know and her specialised duties. The most important requisite to become a midwife was a statement from the parish priest, declaring the applicant to be of good character and a regular churchgoer of unblemished reputation. The reason for this was that, in the women-only situation of childbirth – men weren't permitted into the birthing chamber during the woman's labour – if the child seemed unlikely to survive, it was the midwife's duty to baptise it to enable its soul to enter heaven. An unbaptised baby was denied Christian burial in consecrated ground and was condemned to hell; no one wanted that for the unfortunate infant. Since only women were able to practise midwifery, this was the one and only eventuality where a woman could act as a priest, hence the requirement of a clean reputation and the recommendation of a priest.

In the medieval period and into the eighteenth century, male doctors didn't assist women during childbirth, therefore midwives were indispensable. To some extent, because of their importance, they were able to set their own standards. However, their duties were outlined in Trotula's works and also in Bartholemew's *De Proprietatibus rerum*. This book stated that a midwife should have the craft to assist women in childbirth, in order that they may bear children with less pain and trouble. She should anoint and bathe the mother. She should bathe the child first in water, then in salt and honey to dry up the humours and to comfort his limbs. Then she should wrap him up in swaddling clothes. If the child was sick, she was to use medicines to restore him to health. She should anoint him with noble ointments.

The midwife's task was to safely deliver a mother's unborn child, but also to make things as pleasant for the mother-to-be as possible and to ensure her survival as best she could. During labour, the midwife would rub her patient's belly with a salve to ease her pain and bring her to a quicker parturition. While assuming the sitting or crouching delivery position, usually on a birthing-stool (like a sturdy wooden armchair with a 'U'-shaped cut-out at the front of the seat, so the midwife could ease the baby out with the aid of gravity), the mother would be relaxed by the midwife's comforting words and gestures.

Among the options available to ease the pain of childbirth, none were particularly effective, although some herbal poultices may have eased the discomfort of the contractions just a little. Otherwise, there was always the resort to prayer. Calling upon St Margaret, the patron saint of childbirth, was believed to ease labour pains. According to legend, the saint had stepped out, whole and undamaged, from the belly of the dragon which had swallowed her, and invoking her assistance would therefore ensure a safe delivery. The midwife could assist by rubbing the abdomen of the expectant mother with rose oil, giving her vinegar and sugar to drink, or applying poultices of ivory or eagle's dung.

Gemstones were another possibility. Trotula advised jet as a means of contraception, but magnetic lodestones held in the mother's hand or a coral necklace were believed helpful in relieving the pain of contractions. Hildegard of Bingham also recommended using a stone known as 'sard', a type of chalcedony quartz, similar to carnelian, but darker in colour:

> If a pregnant woman is beset by pain but is unable to give birth, rub sard around both of her thighs and say 'Just as you, O stone, by the order of God, shone on the first angel, so you, child, come forth a shining person, who dwells with God'. Immediately, hold the stone at the exit for the child, that is, the female member, and say 'Open you roads and door in that epiphany by which Christ appeared both human and God, and opened the gates of Hell. Just so, child, may you also come out of this door without dying and without the death of your mother'. Then tie the same stone to a belt and cinch it around her and she will be cured.

Jasper was another gemstone accredited with childbirth-assisting powers. The dried blood of a crane and its right foot were considered useful in labour, but it was this sort of pagan practice that brought midwives into disrepute and ridicule. Another suggestion Hildegard gives for the delivery of a breech birth is that the midwife should 'with her small and gentle hand moistened with a decoction of flaxseed and chickpeas, put the child back in its place and proper position'.

If the delivery of the baby was taking too long, the patient's hair was loosened and all her pins removed. The family or servants would open all doors, drawers, shutters and cupboards in the house and untie any knots, loosen belts and unfasten buckles, in the belief that this helped remove any hindrance to the birth. In cases of difficult births, the mother-to-be could have been advised to put on a holy girdle which would help to alleviate the pains and safeguard her life. Many churches had these birthing girdles carefully stored away and would lend them out to their parishioners – for a fee, of course. Rievaulx Abbey in Yorkshire had a particularly famous girdle. The monks there guarded the girdle of St Ailred, which was known to be particularly helpful to women during their lying-in. If the local church didn't have such an item, you could make your own. *The Sickness of Women*, one of the texts attributed to Trotula, gives instructions for making a beneficial girdle from a hart's (deer's) skin.

Along with the midwife, attending every birth would be the 'gossips', female relatives, friends and neighbours, there to encourage the woman in labour. Their original function had been as 'god-sibs', or godparents, on hand should the baby need immediate baptism. If the labour went on for hours, days even, these women ran out of worthy subjects to talk about and the conversation became more a matter of rumour-mongering and scandal – gossip, in other words.

With the child safely delivered and tended, the placenta (afterbirth) and remains of the detached umbilical cord were burned in the fireplace. One source suggests that the purifying flames were seen as a counterbalance to the sinful means of conception.[18] After the mother was made clean, tidy and presentable, then the father and the rest of the family might be allowed a brief visit to see the newborn in its cradle beside the mother's bed. Then the celebrations could begin. At a few days old, the baby would be paraded to church in procession to be baptised by a priest, with the proud father and designated godparents leading the way, accompanied by the gossips, male family members and neighbours. The mother would remain at home, not allowed to attend church, take the sacraments, touch holy water, bake bread, prepare food or socialise until she had been 'churched'; that is purified and given thanks for her safe delivery, usually six weeks after the birth – one reason why the birthing process is known as a 'confinement'.

Just how far this prohibition against baking bread and preparing food could be observed in a humble home is unknown. In larger, wealthier households, where servants were available to do the cooking, it may well have been possible for the new mother to avoid such tasks, but it seems unlikely that a poor woman could abandon her chores for any length of time, especially if she had other children in her care and a husband demanding his dinner on the table.

Newborn infants were traditionally wrapped in swaddling bands to keep them warm and supported and to encourage their limbs to grow straight. It was believed that the baby's limbs were loosely jointed and any sudden movements might harm his development. In medieval Europe, there were at least two methods of swaddling: the tightly swathed circular technique and the looser criss-cross technique – we don't know which was favoured in England or whether it was a matter of personal preference. Swaddling clothes consisted of a square of cloth with two or more additional bands (like bandages) for securing.[19] Firstly, there may have been a tail-clout (the equivalent of a modern napkin or diaper), tucked between its legs and around its bottom, to help with the three-hourly changing routine, when any soil could be easily removed. The baby was then laid on the swaddling cloth diagonally and the corners were folded over its body and the third up over its feet. The fourth corner padded its head. The bands were wound around and then tied securely. These formed the baby's everyday clothing until it was old enough to sit up and begin moving about, perhaps at six or seven months old.

Unofficial Practitioners

Despite the restrictions, women were active in every community as nurses, midwives and even bonesetters. The famous Paston letters have several references to medical matters. In one letter, dating from 1452, Margaret Paston wrote that her uncle was so ill that he would not survive without medical help, so he was to travel to Suffolk where there was a good physician. On other occasions, and rather more often, the Paston women and their friends themselves acted as healers. For example, in 1455 Alice Crane wrote to Margaret Paston for news of her illness and to ask whether the medicine she had recommended in her last letter had been of any use. There are no details given of Margaret's illness, nor of the contents of the medicine Alice had recommended, which is disappointing, but some letters are more specific.

In Margaret Paston's letter of 1473 to Sir James Gloys, about an illness suffered by her cousin, quite a lot of information was given. It is clear that her cousin had some sort of digestive problem. Margaret suggested that he should use water of mint or water of yarrow (incidentally both these herbs might be prescribed by a herbalist today for digestive problems). She told Sir James that Dame Elesebeth Callethorppe would have either of these waters, and probably others for the same purpose. Dame Elesebeth was obviously known to have store cupboards well stocked with remedies and no doubt there were many people like her. In another letter, Sir John Paston wrote to Dame Margery Paston, asking to have her own special medicine, 'flose ungwentum', to put on a friend's sore knee, and asked her to send him, along with the medicine, directions for how it should be applied and how to store it, whether it should be kept warm, and so on.[20]

It is interesting to see from these references the sort of medical knowledge that the woman of a household might be expected to have. The remedies used by the Pastons and people like them did not differ greatly from many of those recommended in medical texts; for although physicians and surgeons sometimes recommended exotic mixtures containing gold, pearls and expensive spices, they also frequently prescribed mixtures of more homely herbs, lard, honey, eggs and flour. We know that the Paston family owned at least one medical book, which they commissioned a scribe, William Ebesham, to produce for them.

In 1452, Margaret Paston wrote to John Paston asking him for a book with a recipe for chardequince, so that she could take it in the morning as a preventive medicine 'for the air is not wholesome in this town', as she told him. Chardequince was a confection of quinces, honey or sugar, sometimes with other ingredients such as pears and spices. Here is a recipe for chardequince, dated to 1430–50, almost contemporary with Margaret's request (I have modernised the spelling):

> Take a quart of clarified honey, three ounces of powdered pepper and put them together. Take thirty quinces and ten wardens (cooking pears), peal them and draw out the cores and boil them in a good wort* until they are soft. Then pound them in a mortar, adding a little wine if the mixture is too thick, then pass it through a strainer. Put the fruit into the honey and set upon the fire. Let it simmer awhile until it becomes thick but stir it well. Remove it from the fire and add a quarter ounce of powdered ginger, a quarter ounce of galingale and a quarter ounce of cinnamon. Let it cool then put it in a container and sprinkle with ginger and cinnamon.[21]
> [*If wort (a product of brewing) was not available, other recipes say water could be used instead.]

It is interesting that Margaret was planning to make the medicine herself rather than buy it in the town, even though this would mean a delay while her letter was received and the book returned. Recommended as 'a comfort to the stomak', perhaps this was not the sort of remedy that she could expect to buy from an apothecary ready-made, unlike another favourite remedy in times of pestilence, theriac, otherwise known as Venice or Genoa treacle. We looked at theriac in the previous chapter and it is surprising to think this immensely complicated medication, with its many ingredients, could be readily available. Widely recommended in medical texts, we know that ordinary people put their faith in it not only because of the presence in town records of people who made their living by importing and selling it but because the Pastons mention it.

In a letter of 1479, John Paston writes, asking, 'I prey yow send me by the next man that comyth fro London ij pottys of tryacle of Jenne [Genoa] – they shall cost xvj d.' This was urgently required because people were dying in Norwich, where John wrote the letter, and in Swainsthorp where the Pastons had another house, so moving there wasn't an alternative to avoid the sickness. This epidemic was most possibly of plague as treacle was a standard preventive for this.

Chardequince was not the only medicine for everyday problems; many others were simple enough for women like Margaret to concoct in the kitchen, using herbs she could gather from her garden, the fields, hedgerows and woodlands, or else in the spice cupboard. The medieval housewife would store her medications, ready for the time when family, friends or neighbours fell ill. Here are some recipes from a fifteenth-century leechbook, the kind of remedies Margaret might well have made:

Recipe no. 453. A Goode Medecyn for the hede. Take betayn, vverveyne, wormode and celidoyne, weybrede and ruw, walwort and sawge and v cornes of pepper and stamp heme and seth heme togedir in watir and drynke it fastynge. [The ingredients here are betony, vervain, wormwood, greater celandine, greater plantain, rue, ground elder, sage and peppercorns: all readily available.]

Recipe no. 190. Ffor the perilous coughe. Take sawge rw comyn and pepir and seith hem togedir with hony and ete theroff euery day at morrow a sponefull at evyn an other. [Sage, rue, cumin and pepper.]

Recipe no. 197. Ffor a dry cough. Take a garlike hede and rost it at the fire then take away the pyllynge and ete it with good purid hony.

Recipe no. 303. To draw out a splinter. Make an empleyster of southernwood and medle it with fresshe gresse and it will draw owt stubb or thorne that stykkyth in the ffflesshe. [As Dr S. J. Lang reported: 'Unlikely as it may sound, this plaster of southernwood mixed with lard was very effective when I tried it on a large splinter embedded in my finger in the summer of 2005.'][22]

Recipe no. 648. Oyntment for to hele woundis. Take oyle of olyue, hony and may butture of euery ich lich moch and juyse of planteyn as moch as of all tho and seth hem all togedir till that thei be sodden to the haluendelle and then take that ointment and enoynt the wound therwith and it shall hele it faire and clere or elles take lynet and wete therein and lay it in the wound and it shall hele fayre.

Recipe no. 133. Ffor bites and stings. Stamp garlike and lay upon the sore, and for houndis bitynge take hony ther with, and garlyke distroieth venym.

The close relationship between such medicines and cookery is obvious, so no wonder women were perfectly capable of making many remedies in the kitchen. A research project currently underway at Kew Gardens aims to extend our knowledge of British medicinal plants and has already confirmed the usefulness of several of them for exactly the complaints recommended in various herbal remedies.

Whatever the remedies used, whoever administered the treatment, even with the best intentions, things could go wrong. So what happened in such cases when a medical practitioner made a mistake? Taking cases of malpractice and negligence to court is nothing new.

8

MALPRACTICE AND MISBEHAVIOUR – MEDICINE GOES TO COURT

A crooked apothecary can deceive folk well enough on his
   own, but
once he has teamed up with a physician then he can trick
   them
a hundred times over. One writes out the prescription and
   the other
makes it up, yet it costs a florin to buy what is not worth a
   button.

John Gower (*c.* 1330–1408)

As we saw in the previous chapter, in medieval times, many people preferred to consult unofficial medical practitioners, or else took a do-it-yourself approach to treatment when they were unwell. Perhaps the most obvious reason for this was the expense of seeing a professional, or the cost of having them attend you at home. As John Gower tells us in the epigraph above, there was also the fear of being overcharged for the cheapest of medicines. I am sure that the majority of physicians, surgeons and apothecaries, wise women and midwives, were honest enough, just trying to make a living by helping the sick, but it only took one or two cases of fraud and deception to give medical practitioners in general a tarnished reputation. In this chapter, we will explore some of the less reputable aspects of medicine.

Overcharging and Getting Payment

One frequent complaint made against medical practitioners of all kinds concerned the prices they charged for their services. Royal physicians and surgeons could be very well paid. A yearly salary of £40 seems to have been usual during the fourteenth and fifteenth centuries, but £150 wasn't unknown and an extra daily rate was paid on top if the physician or surgeon served the army on campaign abroad. Pancius de Controne was a court physician to both Edward II and Edward III and received £150 per annum at one stage in his career.[1] The Black Prince, eldest son of Edward III, in the mid-fourteenth century, paid his physician, William Blackwater, £40 per annum. When William retired, his pension was even more generous and included a clothing allowance in recognition of the good service he'd given the prince while he was able to work, presumably this being no longer the case.[2]

In the 1360s, William Tankerville, physician to the monks at Westminster Abbey, was being paid in both money and kind by the abbey: £4 a year plus a fur-trimmed robe befitting his profession at a cost of 26s 8d. In the accounts of 1368–69, his clothing allowance was raised to 30s 4d, so that he could have a robe 'with three furs'.[3] Was that a particularly cold winter and the monks didn't want their physician going down with a chill when they were most in need of his services? This expensive robe may have been of the traditional colours of red and grey. William Langland, in his work *The Vision of Piers Plowman*, described a physician with his furred hood and his fine cloak decorated with gold buttons.[4] This is Geoffrey Chaucer's description of the Doctor in the prologue to his *Canterbury Tales*, wearing fine robes and coveting money:

In blood-red garments, slashed with bluish grey
And lined with taffeta, he rode his way;
Yet he was rather close as to expenses
And kept the gold he won in pestilences.[5]

This was another common assumption about medieval practitioners
– that they thrived on the misfortunes of others, especially during
the epidemics that they wished for, as in this excerpt from
Chaucer's *The Romaunt of the Rose*:

They would that forty were sick at once,
Ye, two hundred, in flesh and bones,
And yet two thousand, as I guess,
For to increase their riches.
They will not work in any way
But for money and covetousness.[6]

Judging from the goods, chattels and bequests left in the wills
of various practitioners, their business could be very lucrative.
Nicholas Colnet was a physician who served Henry V during the
Agincourt campaign of 1415. He wrote his will before he again
attended the king in France, in 1417, and died three years later,
in November 1420. His bequests added up to more than £115 in
money, in addition to lavish gifts of silver and gilt plate, fine cloth
and jewellery. He was generous to Bethlehem Hospital, just outside
London, and to his two sisters, his brother and a niece.[7] Receiving
such fees and payment in kind, like the gold and ruby ring given
by the Duchess of Norfolk to the physician Walter Leinster for a
successful cure,[8] is it any wonder people were wary that they too
might be overcharged for their medical treatment?

In 1408, John Luter, described as a leech of London, was
ordered to appear before the Lord Mayor, Drew Barentyn. Luter's
patient, John Clotes, accused the physician of not only charging

him an exorbitant fee but also of failing to cure him. Clotes had given Luter fifteen semi-precious stones called 'serpentynes' worth 9 marks, a gold tablet worth £3 and a sword costing 6s 8d. These valuables were to be kept by the physician only if the treatment was successful. Since this hadn't happened, the patient wanted his goods returned. Luter argued that he was entitled to keep everything because Clotes had asked to be cured of 'salsefleume', a scabrous skin problem. When it became clear to the physician that he actually had leprosy, which was incurable, he claimed that he had already incurred costs and had taught the patient how to make himself a balsam treatment and other medications, so the fee had been well earned, despite the failure to cure. However, Drew Barentyne found in the patient's favour; Luter had received the valuables 'fraudulently, deceptively and injuriously' and lost the case.[9]

Not all royal physicians were so well paid and not all physicians overcharged. Dominic de Sergio, whom we met earlier in chapter 4, wasn't always paid on time by his royal employer, Edward IV. Although promised an annuity of £40 every year in 1471, Sergio had yet to be paid at all in 1475, despite constant pleas to the Exchequer. A token remittance was eventually forthcoming, but he was still owed £100 when he disappeared from the records that year, having received £53 6s 8d 'for good service to the King, his consort and daughters'. John Crophill of Wix in Essex, whom we met in chapter 3, was treating his humble patients, the carpenter, the cordwainer, the herdsman and the sexton, for a few pence a time, making good his losses by charging his wealthier patients rather more. In Belstone village, William Fortlie paid just 2d while Richard Armystyd paid 6s 8d and John Armystyd paid 13s 4d, the Armystyd family being among the more affluent inhabitants of Otley.[10] Friar Thomas Stanfield could afford to give him a set of drinking cups with which Crophill seems to have wooed a number of ladies of Wix. This was the accepted method of making the job pay at the time, as was the practice of prescribing cheap medicines for the poor and more elaborate ones for the rich. For example, a laxative suitable for the wealthy was a triple infusion of rhubarb – at the time an exotic foreign import – but for the poor it was simply 'plums', although they were probably just as effective. Similarly, it was recommended that nasty-looking medicines should be gilded with gold leaf before being administered to a rich patient; giving the same to a poor patient was advisedly done in the dark and drunk through a straw from a narrow-necked bottle.[11]

A case in London from 1320 shows how determined some medical men were to get their fee. The surgeon John of Cornhill was summoned to answer an accusation of trespass made by Alice of Stockynge, a patient of his in Fleet Street. Alice had a problem with her feet and John visited her at home, promising a cure within a fortnight. However, after less than a week of his treatment with 'diverse medicaments', she couldn't put her feet to the floor and the infirmity was now reckoned to be incurable. Denied his fee, John forced his way into Alice's house and stole a blanket, two sheets and a tunic worth twenty shillings. In court, he denied ever promising to cure Alice or using medications that had infected her feet and said he had certainly not entered her house against her will. Despite his claims, the jury believed otherwise and found in Alice's favour, awarding her the considerable sum of £30 16s 8d in damages against the surgeon.[12] The amount of damages awarded here probably reflects the fact that this wasn't just about demanding payment in an illegal manner, but also dealt with the fact that the treatment had made the patient much worse, possibly incurable – a case of malpractice.

Malpractice and Negligence

Whether or not medical professionals were generally charging too highly for their work, a far more serious possibility for the patient was if the doctor got things wrong. This wasn't just a matter of making a mistake in the treatment carried out, but might be a case of conducting the correct procedure at the wrong time. We saw in chapter 5 how important astrology was to the practice of medicine, with Zodiac Men being used regularly to determine when it was safe to treat a patient's particular problem. In 1424, a lawsuit was brought against a London surgeon, John Harwe, and two barber-surgeons, John Dalton and Simon Rolf, who had treated William Forset (or Forest) in an emergency for a wounded hand. On 31 January, with the moon in the 'bloody' sign of Aquarius 'under a very malevolent constellation', William had severely injured his right thumb. There is no mention of him seeking medical help immediately, but on 9 February, with the moon now in Gemini, the sign with dominion over the arms and hands, William's thumb bled profusely. Simon Rolf managed to staunch the bleeding temporarily, then John Harwe, assisted by John Dalton, stopped the bleeding. But, the record says, 'it [the bleeding] broke out six several times in a dangerous fashion'. Eventually, with the patient's permission when his life seemed in danger, Harwe cauterised the wound 'as was proper' and saved William's life. But now, the patient wanted the surgeon and his fellows to pay damages because the muscles of his thumb were no longer functioning properly, claiming they shouldn't have treated him when the astrological aspects were all against it.[13]

Eight reputable physicians and surgeons of London, including Gilbert Kymer, Thomas Morstede and William Bradwardyne, sat in judgement on the case. They concluded that the three defendants had acted in the surgically correct manner and had made no error. William's problems, mutilation and disfigurement of his hand were caused by a) the situation of the constellations on the day of the original injury, b) by the same on the day he had to seek treatment, or c) some defect in the patient himself. Whatever the case, the adjudicators said, the defendants were guiltless and had been maliciously defamed, undeservedly damaging their good reputations. William Forset was to keep silent on the matter and withdraw all charges against them.

In London, a case was brought against the surgeon Richard Cheyndut by the son of Walter de Hull, one of Cheyndut's patients. In 1377, Walter suffered 'a malady' of his left leg. Whatever kind of treatment Cheyndut administered, it made matters worse rather than better. On the mayor's instruction, three surgeons examined Walter's leg and determined that only 'great experience, great care and great expense' could possibly have prevented further, permanent injury to his limb. In the event, Cheyndut was fined the huge sum of 50s in damages and spent a term in gaol as well.[14]

There was an occasion in York, in 1433, when the Prior of Guisborough and one of his monks, Brother Richard, tried to sue Matthew Rillesford, a practising leech in York, for £40 damages. Matthew had become a freeman of the city three years earlier, being described as a *medicus*, a Latin term for a physician, yet it seems he didn't have any university education nor a licence to practise. Perhaps that was the reason why, instead of taking the case to a court of law, the parties agreed to the arbitration of an experienced apothecary, Robert Belton of York.[15]

Brother Richard had injured his left tibia, maybe broken it, and Matthew had promised to cure it, they said, but instead Richard's whole body had become infected. Matthew claimed that he had never said he would cure the monk. Brother Richard complained that in applying the so-called cure Matthew had been negligent in his treatment, making him far worse. Matthew responded that it was the monk's own fault because he continued to eat the unwholesome food Matthew had forbidden as part of the treatment, hindering the effectiveness of the medicine and bringing on a bout of diarrhoea. Having heard both sides of the argument, Robert Belton adjudicated that Matthew had to be given eight days to bring about Richard's cure, applying his medicines under Robert's personal supervision. Until then, the prior and the monk were to suspend any action against Matthew. Since the records show nothing more on the matter, we may assume that Brother Richard's leg was healed.

By a London ordinance of 1416, a medical practitioner could be heavily fined if he failed to inform the authorities – the relevant guild masters or the lord mayor's office – within four days that he was treating a case so severe it might well result in the patient's death or mutilation of some kind. The intention was that the practitioner should consult with his colleagues and be advised by his peers on the proposed treatments, in order to guard against such malpractice suits. In 1435, the fine for not reporting and consulting on dangerous cases was set at 13s 4d. The ordinance was a safeguard for the patient against reckless and unconsidered treatment by the doctor, as well as a means of defending the profession against the possibilities of damning prosecutions.

To cover themselves, surgeons had to pay a kind of medieval insurance premium to the mayor's office, a recognisance, when they took on a high-risk patient, in case it resulted in a malpractice suit. In 1417, the surgeon John Severell Love was recorded as owing the chamberlain of London 20s for his recognisance. If he informed the authorities as required whenever he took on a critical patient, the money would remain untouched, but if he failed to alert them within the specified four days and the patient or the patient's family sued him in the courts, the money was forfeit: half to the city and half to the craft of surgeons.[16] What is unclear is whether all London practitioners were required to pay this recognisance in advance of accepting any patients, high risk or otherwise. It seems unlikely that those starting out on their career could readily afford such a large sum of 20s, or maybe there was a sliding scale for recognisance, depending on the practitioner's standing in the guild and his likelihood of taking on a patient with little chance of making a good recovery. After all, the medical books warned against accepting cases that would do nothing to enhance the doctor's reputation. A dead or maimed patient was a poor advertisement for any professional although, in the event of a recovery against the odds, that would do wonders for the practitioner's standing in the community – such matters had to be taken into consideration.

Whatever precautions were taken to guard against possible malpractice on the part of professional physicians and surgeons, there was no certain protection against the actions of those who might masquerade as bona fide practitioners, but were nothing of the kind. In 1376, Roger Clerk of Wandelsworth (Wandsworth) was summoned to appear before the Mayor of London on a charge that no physician or surgeon in the city 'should intermeddle with medicines or cures unless experienced and licensed therein'. Roger Clerk had received no training and was illiterate yet he had attended Roger atte Hache's wife, Johanna, who was ill with 'certain bodily infirmities' and a fever. Atte Hache gave Clerk 12*d* in advance for treatment with the balance to be paid when Johanna recovered. Clerk rolled a piece of tattered old parchment inside a scrap of cloth of gold and hung it around her neck, assuring the patient that it would heal her ailments and banish her fever. The cure didn't work and her husband took Clerk to court, accusing him as a false physician. This was a serious matter, not just because Clerk had misled atte Hache and his wife, but because he was subsequently regarded by the mayor and aldermen as a threat to the whole population of London with his deceitful misrepresentation.

In court, Clerk maintained that the piece of parchment was an amulet, inscribed with a sacred text in Latin. This he recited before the assembly, a sure treatment for the patient's ills, so he claimed:

Anima Christi, sanctifica me; corpus Christi, salve me; in isanguis Christi, nebria me; cum bonus Christi tu, lave me.

The first two phrases mean something like 'Soul of Christ, sanctify me; body of Christ, save me'. The third phrase doesn't make sense

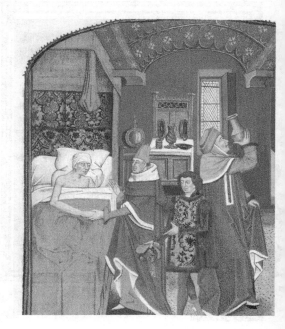

Right: 1. Vespasian suffering from leprosy and being examined in bed by two doctors. From Eustache Marcadé, *Mystère de la Vengeance de Nostre Seigneur Ihesu Crist*, Burgundy France, 1465.

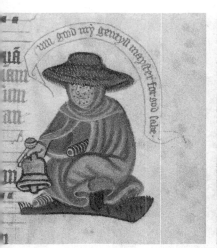

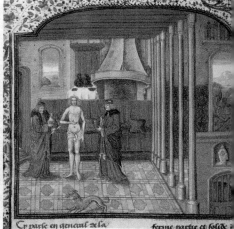

Above left: 2. Leper with bell. Pontifical Tabular, England, early fifteenth century.

Above right: 3. Patient with saints Cosmas and Damian. From Bartholomaeus Anglicus, *De proprietatibus rerum*, Bruges, 1482.

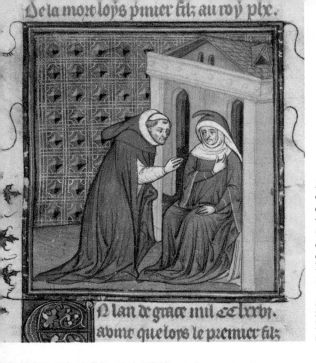

De la mox loys pinier fili; au roy ple.

N lan de grace mil cc lxxbi.
abint que loys le premier fili;

Left: 4. Abbot of Saint Denis consulting a wise-woman. *Chroniques de France ou de St Denis*, France, about 1300.

cc(xxvi

Below: 5. Stones of Rhodes and snake stones.

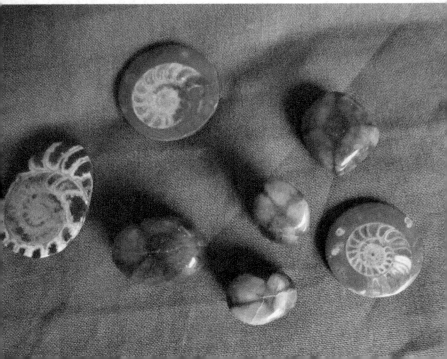

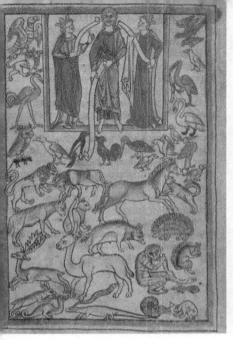

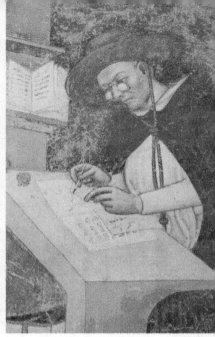

Above left: 6. Adam naming the animals. Northumberland Bestiary, England, about 1250.

Above right: 7. First illustration of spectacles. Cardinal Hugh of Saint Claire (Hugh de Provence) in a fresco by Tomaso of Modena, Italy, 1352.

Below: 7a. Monks wearing spectacles at Archeon Living History Museum, Netherlands.

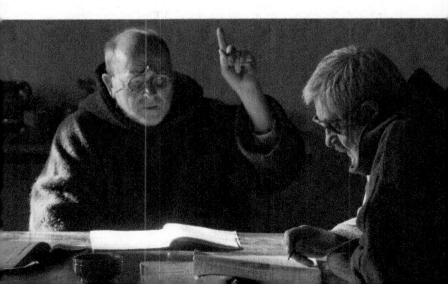

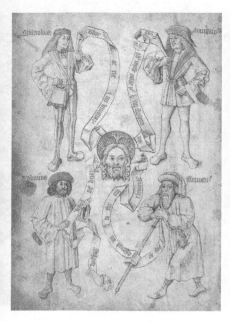

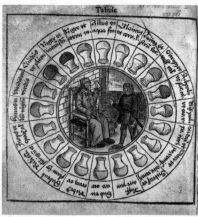

Left: 8. The Four Humours. From the Guild Book of the Barber Surgeons of York, England, about 1486.

Above: 9. Urine colour chart. From Ulrich Pinder, *Epiphaniae medicorum*, Nuremberg, Germany, about 1510.

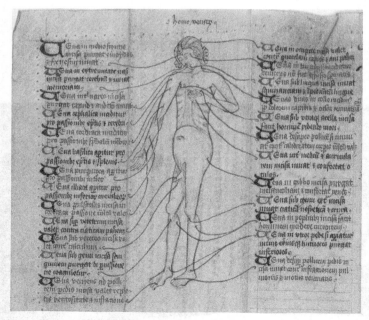

10. Vein Man. From the Folding Almanac, England, late fifteenth century.

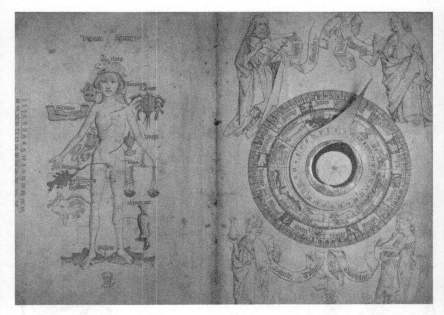

11. Zodiac man and a volvelle (incomplete). From the Guild Book of the Barber Surgeons of York, England, about 1486.

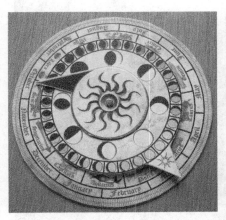

Above: 11a. Reproduction volvelle.

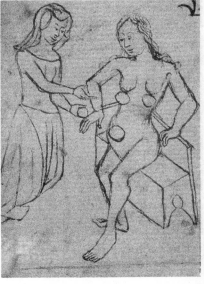

Right: 12. Female surgeon cupping a female patient. From a medical treatise by John of Arderne, England, mid-fifteenth century.

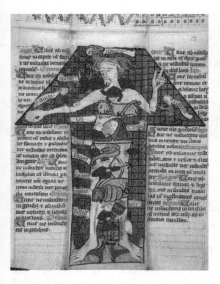

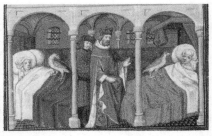

Left: 13. Zodiac Man. The man's pointing finger serves as a warning against the powerful forces of the stars' astrology. From a physician's folding calendar, England, early fifteenth century.

Above: 14. Caladrius bird in action. From the Talbot Shrewsbury Book, France, 1145.

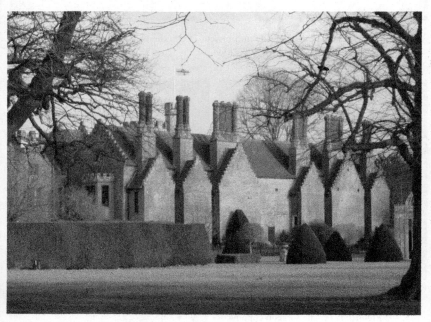

15. Chenies Manor, Amersham, Buckinghamshire, showing its windowless face to the miasmas of London.

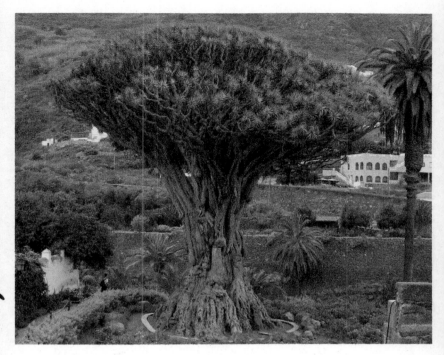

16. Dragon's blood tree (*Dracaena draco*) in Tenerife.

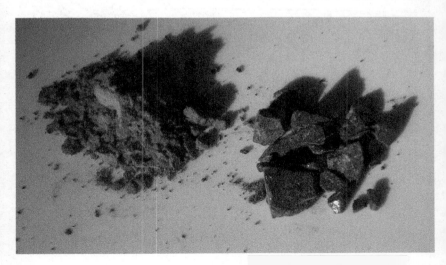

16a. Dragon's blood resin.

Dragon's Blood resin

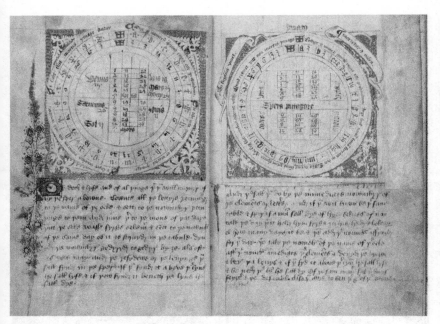

17. Spheres of Pythagoras. From A Physician's Handbook, England, about 1454.

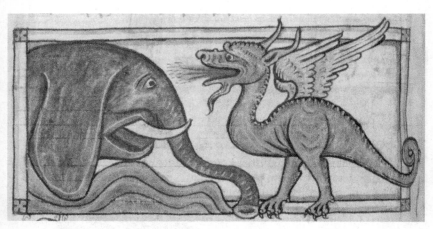

18. Elephant and a dragon. From an English bestiary, about 1250.

Right: 19. Mandrake. From Jacob Meydenbach, *Hortus Sanitatis* (*Garden of Health*), Germany, 1491.

Below left: 20. Dame Trotula, empress among midwives. France, early fourteenth century.

Below right: 21. Jar for Mithridate and Theriac. Italian, about 1580.

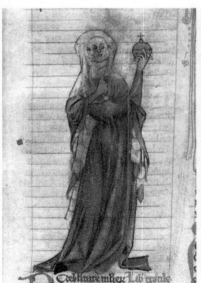

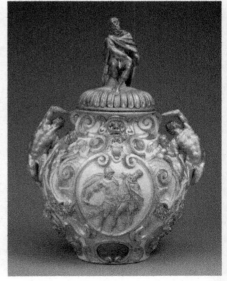

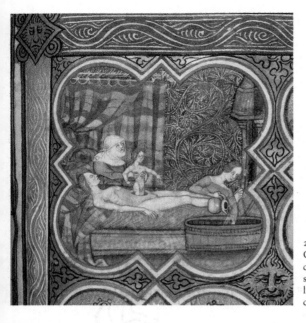

22. Birth of
Caesar by
caesarean
section. France,
late fourteenth
century.

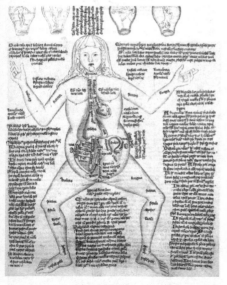

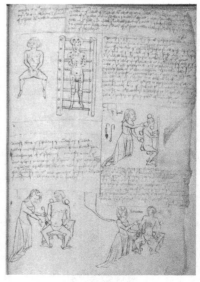

Above left: 23. Pregnant woman with possible positions of the foetus. From *The Apocalypse of St John*, Germany, 1420.

Above right: 24. Female surgeon. From John Arderne's treatise, England, *c.* 1425.

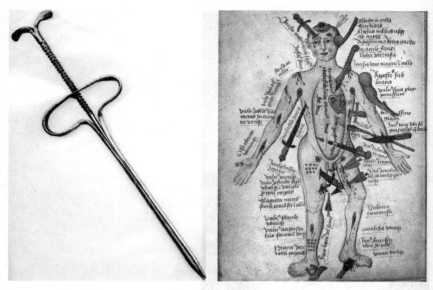

Above left: 25. Modern replica of John Bradmore's instrument.

Above right: 26. Wound Man. From *Anathomia*, England, mid-fifteenth century.

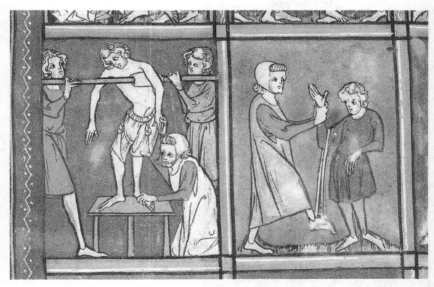

27. Surgeon treating patients with broken or dislocated bones. By Roger Frugard of Parma, France, early fourteenth century.

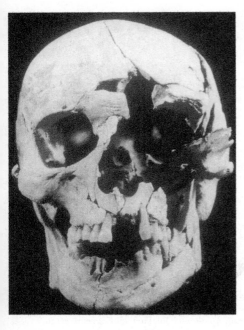

28. Towton 16 skull.

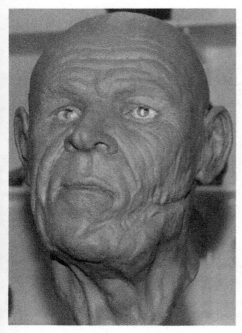

28a. Towton 16 facial reconstruction.

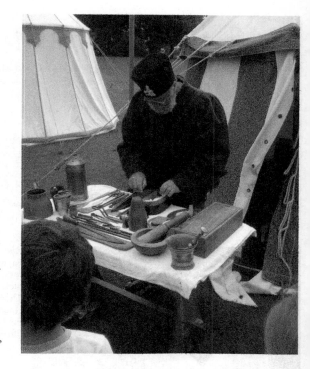

Right: 29.
Medieval barber-
surgeon at
Rochester Castle.

Below: 29a.
Disabled beggar
in buggy at
Archeon Living
History Museum,
Netherlands.

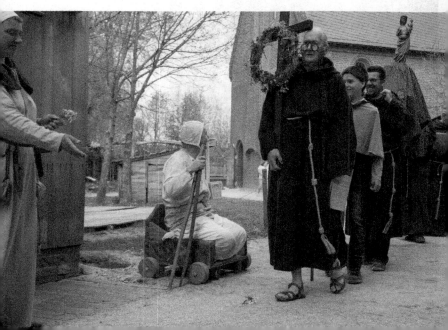

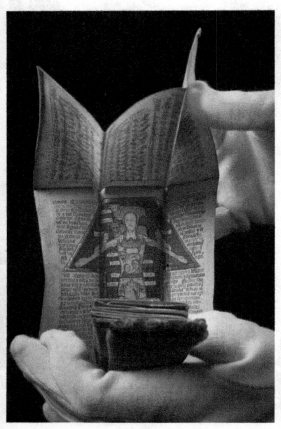

Above: 30. Thomas Fayreford's charm for staunching blood. From Thomas Fayreford's commonplace book, England, early fifteenth century.

Left: 31. English folding almanac. England, 1415.

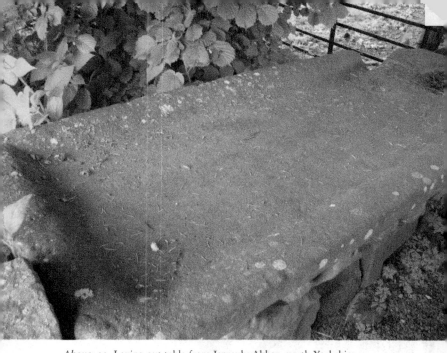

Above: 32. Laying-out table from Jervaulx Abbey, north Yorkshire.

Below: 33. An alchemist at work at Archeon Living History Museum, Netherlands.

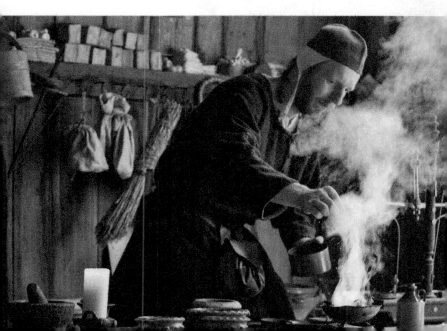

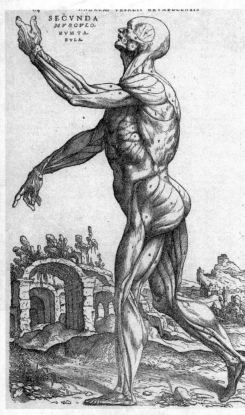

34. A page from *De humani corporis fabrica* by Versalius, 1514–64.

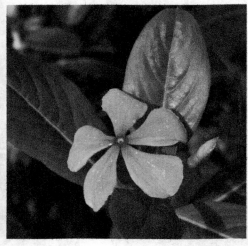

35. Madagascan or rosy periwinkle (*Catharanthus roseus*).

(obviously Clerk wasn't even very skilled at learning by rote) – it might have been intended to be *in sanguis Christi, inebria me*, or similar: 'in Christ's blood, drench me' – and ends 'with thy goodness Christ, wash me'. The grammar is poor but this is probably what was meant, if anything had actually been written on the parchment. However, when the parchment was examined, there was no sacred text, just a few illiterate scratches. Clerk was convicted of being an imposter, utterly ignorant of the medicinal arts and therefore a danger to the community that might seek his assistance in future. To guard against this, Clerk's humiliating punishment was to be carried out in full view of the citizens, to ensure that they would know of his deceitful charade, as well as acting as a deterrent to any other would-be dubious practitioners without education or training. He was led on a rope through the centre of the city by a man on horseback, with trumpeters and pipers playing to attract attention. The parchment scrap, a whetstone and two urine flasks – the universal symbols of physicians – were hung around his neck so all would understand his crime.[17]

Even more spurious was the case of John Crok in 1371. The king's justices in the civil courts in London ordered Crok to present himself before them and to bring his bag for examination – the bag having been rumoured to contain a dead man's head. Crok brought his bag, as demanded, and explained that it was the head of a Saracen that he'd bought in Toledo in Spain. He needed it as a container to house a spirit, so that he could ask it questions: the ears would hear and the mouth would answer. There was also a book in the bag which contained explanations and experiments, but Crok insisted that he hadn't used either the head or the book. Nevertheless, his bag and the contents were burned in the presence of King Edward III at Westminster and Crok was forced to swear on the gospels that he wouldn't do anything else 'contrary to faith' ever again.[18]

Another problem for the city authorities in London was that of men from elsewhere who, although qualified, weren't licensed to practise medicine there, nor were they members of the appropriate guilds. Apart from robbing the local doctors of patients – a scandal in itself – there was the fear of 'damage, deceit and abuses' by these 'rebellious' practitioners who were arriving daily from 'the sticks'. That was the term used to describe incomers, especially those from distant parts of England. Wardens were appointed to examine these newcomers to the city who were not to be granted a licence until they had proven themselves 'good and able'; otherwise, they were to be fined 40*d*.

One last malpractice case is worth mentioning since it happened in 'the sticks' of Devon and was brought against Pernell, who is described as 'a woman physician', alongside her husband, Thomas de Rasyn, also a physician. The pair was accused of causing the death of a miller in Sidmouth because of their ignorance and poor practices. Found guilty on 7 August 1350, they were made outlaws. Banished from home and with assistance of any kind from anyone forbidden, this was a virtual death sentence. But Pernell and Thomas did not give in: they appealed to the Crown and received a royal pardon and the reinstatement of their reputations.[19] This was quite an exceptional outcome.

Misbehaviour

Physicians and surgeons were expected to be pillars of the community, after all; they attended people at their most vulnerable, and if you couldn't trust the doctor then who could you rely on? For this reason, medical men were required to be respectable and beyond reproach and the Companies of Surgeons, the Guilds of Barber-Surgeons and Colleges of Physicians across the country and on the Continent demanded that their members' behaviour should never bring the associations, of whatever kind, into disrepute. That was the ideal, but medical practitioners were only human. In 1474, in the reign of Edward IV, a London barber-surgeon named

John Denys was arrested and brought before the lord mayor and aldermen on a charge of bawdry. Today, we would call it pimping. The case resulted in Denys's imprisonment, but he appealed to the Chancery Court, which dealt with financial prosecutions, presumably on the grounds of a loss of earnings while he was in prison and, maybe, the likelihood of a reduced income after his release because of the stain on his reputation. There was also the possibility that his regular patients had had to take their problems to some other barber-surgeon in the meantime and might not return to him. In answer to a writ from Chancery, the mayor had to defend his actions in arresting and imprisoning Denys. By the later fifteenth century, such correspondence was usually written in English, but in this case the gravity of the matter required a bit of Latin to give it emphasis. It translates as:

Just as crows and eagles, by the instinct of their nature, converge where dead bodies lie, so also do bawds attract to their bawdy-houses, by their nefarious vice of lust, other evildoers, whence comes murder, robbery, felonies, litigiousness, dissensions and other evil deeds against the king's peace and the healthy and politic rule of the kingdom.[20]

It was always assumed that bawdy houses weren't just palaces of prostitution, but the hideouts of the criminal class where all manner of wicked deeds were conceived and planned. The people who ran these dens of iniquity were often in trouble with the authorities, but in Denys's case it seems they took it to the full letter of the law. The Guild of Barber-Surgeons would have had an interest too. Clearly, there was no chance of keeping things under wraps, so the alternative was to let the public see justice being done, the proof that a medical man who brought the profession into disrepute would suffer the consequences. This was necessary to maintain public trust.

Another medical man who brought disgrace upon himself and his profession was the royal physician and surgeon William Hobbys, whom we met earlier. William had been married to his wife Alice for twenty years and they had five children. While in France, serving on campaign with King Edward IV, in the summer of 1475, his fellow surgeons, Richard Chamber and John Staveley – Staveley happened to be Hobbys's son-in-law, wedded to his daughter, Mercy – had noticed William sneaking off to the local brothels in the evenings. Chamber said he'd seen his colleague lying in bed, naked, with a prostitute in the village of Péronne in Picardy, and had spoken with him, incredulous at such misbehaviour. Staveley reported that his father-in-law had visited brothels on numerous occasions during the French campaign, in Calais and Saint-Omer, as well as Péronne, 'to commit adultery', he said.

Hobbys's misconduct abroad was not just a case of enjoying himself while away from home. He later admitted that it had been his habit to visit prostitutes in London and Southwark since 1462, sleeping with and committing adultery with 'many different women'. In June 1474, Robert Halyday, Master of the Guild of Barber-Surgeons, and his colleague Thomas Rolf were called urgently to attend a brothel keeper who had been seriously injured in a fight at a Southwark stew. Having tended the patient, the surgeons happened to glance through a spyhole in the wall into the next cubicle and saw William Hobbys in the arms of a pretty young prostitute. Halyday was shocked and in his capacity as guild master, confronted Hobbys, gave him a good telling off for not only cheating on his wife, Alice, but bringing the good name of the guild into disrepute. If he didn't mend his ways, they threatened to tell Alice. The threats had no effect, but Halyday wasn't bluffing, although it seems Hobbys was given at least a year's grace.

Sometime before Christmas 1475, after the French expedition, when it had become obvious that he wasn't going to reform, they finally told Hobbys's wife, Alice. She claimed she had no idea of her husband's adultery in all those years of marriage. In 1476, she brought a case against him, in the Church court held in St Paul's Cathedral, for violating the matrimonial bed by committing adultery. The court found in her favour; henceforth she would not be required 'to consort or cohabit with the said William, nor to render the conjugal debt' (i.e. he could no longer demand his marital right to have sex with her). It was incredibly rare for a husband's adultery to be considered such a serious breach of canon law. Out of 250 cases of adultery recorded in this particular document at the London Metropolitan Archive, this is the only one that resulted in the legal separation of spouses.[21] It would seem that both the Church authorities and the Guild of Barber-Surgeons intended to make an example of Hobbys, not only to demonstrate that such misbehaviour on the part of a professional would not be tolerated but also to restore public faith in the medical fraternity as a whole. Divorce was never an option in medieval England, but Alice was granted permission to quit her husband's 'bed and board', although neither was free to marry again.[22]

Surprisingly, the case doesn't seem to have done Hobbys any damage with regard to his career. He continued to serve as King Edward's physician and surgeon and was employed by King Richard III in the same office. It is possible, judging by the tone of his will, proven in 1488, that he became a reformed character after the separation from Alice, taking religion far more seriously, 'trusting in the Blessed Mary ... and all the saints ... and thus I trust in them against all the shackles of demons'.[23]

Forensic Medicine

Perhaps not quite what we've come to expect of forensic scientists as seen on TV, or read about in crime thrillers, but medieval practitioners were occasionally called to the scene of a suspicious death or summoned as expert witnesses in court. In 1281, in Venice, a law was passed requiring physicians and surgeons to report all cases of serious wounding or unexplained deaths to the authorities, as well as notifying them of any cases of leprosy. England did not have such a law, but the coroners had the power to call upon the medical profession as and when needed to determine the cause of death or, in the case of an inflicted traumatic injury, whether this was likely to prove fatal within the specified period of a year and a day, in which case it would be murder. The Church also required expert medical testimony regarding the alleged miracles of healing performed by any would-be saint, as part of the official process of canonisation.

Today's forensic evidence is often acquired through detailed post-mortem procedures but, because the Church ruled against human dissection, in medieval times the examination of a corpse was mostly limited to what could be seen on the outside. Even if internal examination had been permitted, it seems likely that only the most obvious trauma would have been apparent, since the practitioners of the time had so little knowledge as to the 'normal' appearance of human organs, necessary to be able to make a considered comparison.

One possible problem that might confront a doctor in any period of history was to determine whether a body was devoid of life or simply deeply unconscious. As examples, there are at least two modern incidents where, despite modern medical technology, a 'body' turned out to be still alive. Fijian-born Derek Derenalagi joined the British Army and was serving a tour of duty in Helmand Province in Afghanistan in July 2007 when his vehicle was blown up by an improvised explosive device (IED). Back at Camp Bastion he was pronounced dead, but while preparing his body for a body bag medical staff found that he still had a pulse. As a result of the injuries he sustained, both Derenalagi's legs were amputated above the knee. In a coma, he was flown back to the UK where, nine days later, he woke up in hospital, in Birmingham. He has since become a British Paralympic discus thrower.[24]

The second case is that of Walter Williams, a seventy-nine-year-old Mississippi farmer. In February 2014 he went into a hospice suffering from congestive heart failure. On 27 February he was pronounced dead; nurses, doctors and a coroner having searched for and failed to find a pulse. He was put into a body bag and transferred to a funeral home. When he began stirring and rustling inside the bag, incredulous staff called an ambulance to take Walter back to the hospice where he survived for another three weeks.[25] Evidently mistakes can still be made, so what did medieval practitioners do to ensure the body was truly dead?

There were a number of tests that could be tried, and, although none of them could have been absolutely certain, taken together they would have given little cause for doubt. Inflicting 'deep pain', such as the doctor grinding his knuckles into the patient's sternum (breast bone) or crushing his fingernail bed between two hard objects – a bit like thumbscrews – would have been sufficient to rouse the deepest sleeper. Unconsciousness caused by trauma or drug-induced by sleeping potions would need more detailed examination.

A thirteenth-century manuscript, dated to around 1280, Ashmole MS 399 in the Bodleian Library in Oxford, has a series of pictures (ff.33r–34r) showing a physician treating a woman from her first collapse throughout her illness and death. At this point he hands over to a barber-surgeon, wielding a knife for the post-mortem and displaying her internal organs. In one image, the physician is burning a feather beneath her nose to revive her – the medieval equivalent of smelling salts – then, in f.33v, he is seen balancing a dish of water on the patient's chest, such that any rippling of the surface would demonstrate that she was still breathing.

In other cases, the eyes would have been a good indicator. On opening the eyelid, the pupil should first constrict as the light hits it and then dilate a little as it gauges the level of brightness and settles – indoors or at night, the medieval doctor would have needed a good quality candle for this. Overly dilated or constricted pupils may have suggested an overdose of some drug or other. If the pupils didn't react similarly, this would have indicated trauma to the brain, such as a concussion or a stroke[26] – an apoplexy was the medieval term. If the pupils failed to react at all, if touching the eyeball initiated no response, then it was time to hand over the patient to a priest.

Into the early modern period, perhaps from 1550 onwards, at a time when women were being increasingly confined to domestic matters, midwives were bucking the trend. One of the few public positions open to women, midwifery allowed them to carry out a variety of duties in the community. Town councils, especially in Europe, now employed official midwives, mainly to supervise the deliveries of poor women, as part of their social care policies. Midwives were also asked to oversee moral standards and report on pregnancies among unmarried women. In addition, they were expected to give expert testimony in court in legal cases involving a female body, such as rape cases and claims involving men who were reckoned not to have 'de-flowered' their brides.

A case from York in 1432 involved both midwives and prostitutes in their official capacities. Alice Russell, aged twenty-six, had been wed to John Skathelok for more than two years and, so Alice claimed, John had yet 'to know her carnally'. Joan Semer, a forty-year-old woman of 'free status and good standing' gave testimony in court to the same effect. She also declared that Alice was 'well formed, strong and willing to be a mother', if only her husband was sufficiently potent. It seems likely that Joan was a licensed midwife since she had examined Alice, although the report doesn't actually state her profession. The other nine women involved in giving evidence were prostitutes. They had come together with John – he with his hose and breeches unfastened and taken down to his knees – and the women did all they could to rouse his penis to become erect. They kissed him, fondled him and let him touch them intimately, but there was no response. The report, written in Latin, gives details of everything the women tried. The court found in Alice's favour and dissolved the marriage on the grounds of poor John's impotence and she was free to take a new husband.[27]

In cases of alleged infanticide, midwives were asked to inspect the defendant's body and testify as to whether or not she had recently given birth. This happened in Eton, near Windsor, in 1517. Alice Ridyng was accused of having suffocated her newborn baby boy when he was just a few hours old and buried him in the dungheap in her father's orchard. Alice hadn't told anyone that she was pregnant and nobody had been with her during the birth, but 'some women of Windsor and Eton had suspected' despite Alice denying it, insisting that 'something else was wrong with her belly'. The child was born on a Sunday and on the Tuesday 'the honest [mid]wives took her and inspected her belly and her breasts by which they knew for certain that she had given birth'. Alice then confessed that her parents had known nothing and swore on the gospels that only Thomas Denys, the chaplain at a nearby infirmary, had lain with her carnally. She also admitted that no one had urged or agreed to the baby being killed.[28] Whether or how she was punished isn't recorded, but this is another example of midwives being involved as 'expert witnesses' in court cases.

Taking Advantage

As we have seen, there were medical men who broke the rules, from overcharging the patient to blatant deception by unqualified charlatans, from immorality to negligence. But perhaps one of the worst transgressions was that of using the position of professional and personal trust to perpetrate acts of treason. In the summer of 1483, the Welsh physician, mathematician and astrologer Lewis Caerleon did just that.

With King Richard III newly seated upon his uneasy throne, Margaret Beaufort, mother of Henry Tudor, was busy plotting the return of her son from exile with a view to displacing Richard. Claiming ill health, Margaret employed the services of Caerleon, seeking his advice on medical matters and much more besides. She intended that her son, Henry Tudor, should marry the late

King Edward's eldest daughter, thus uniting the warring houses of York and Lancaster, in order to give Henry's attempt at seizing the throne more support. His claim was otherwise spurious to say the least. The proposed marriage had to be discussed with the late king's widow, Elizabeth Woodville, but this proved difficult with the widow keeping herself and her children in sanctuary in Westminster Abbey. However, Margaret was a determined and artful woman. Medical men, by the nature of their profession, could come and go openly, even into sanctuary, without causing suspicion. Margaret needed a go-between who was sufficiently respected and above reproach, so that he might move freely between the two women, carrying their treasonous correspondence. It was arranged that Caerleon would visit the widow under the guise of tending her health while actually engaged in hatching a treasonous conspiracy, raising a rebellion on behalf of Margaret's son.[29]

Matters didn't quite work out as they'd planned. This time around, the rebellion failed miserably and Lewis Caerleon was arrested by King Richard, who seized all his possessions and had him imprisoned in the Tower of London. Despite the significant role he had played in the conspiracy, Caerleon wasn't executed for treason, but was permitted to spend his time in the Tower writing an astrological treatise. Whether his deliberations successfully forecast the future or not, we cannot tell, but if they did, Caerleon would have known that Henry Tudor's next attempt at deposing King Richard would result in a resounding victory. Caerleon would profit handsomely for his treasonous services to Margaret with his promotion to the post of royal physician and a fee of 60 marks a year. He would attend the new Tudor king, Henry VII, and his queen, Elizabeth of York, whose marriage he had helped devise. But before that, Henry had to defeat King Richard at the Battle of Bosworth on 22 August 1485, which brings us to the subject of the next chapter: medicine on the battlefield.

9

MEDICINE ON THE
BATTLEFIELD

[Surgery] rests most principally in manual application of
   medicines,
in staunching of blood, searching of wounds with iron and
   other instruments,
in cutting of the skull ... taking out bones, sewing of flesh ...
with other suchlike ... in manual operation.
                    From Thomas Ross's *Definition of Surgery*, 1519

Medieval battles were brutal and bloody. Depending on the
era, mounted knights in chainmail or plate armour, armed with
lances, morning stars and maces, charged at men-at-arms wielding
swords, pikes and battleaxes, all of them subject to hailstorms of
arrows, cannon shot and, towards the end of our period, gunfire.
Unavoidably, there were numerous casualties. Those who were
killed outright were probably the lucky ones, for a nasty wound
might mean a slow and painful death. For those who were
unfortunate enough to suffer more than the inevitable minor cuts
and bruises, what could the surgeons do for them and what were
the chances of long-term survival and recovery? Surprisingly, their
chances might have been better than you think.

King Richard the Lionheart

One battlefield casualty who didn't survive, despite having the best treatment available at the time, was King Richard I, known as the Lionheart. Although he was more French than English in every way, Richard had actually been born in England on 8 September 1157 at Castle Beaumont, Oxford. He became king in 1189 and immediately made plans to go on Crusade to the Holy Land. In his reign of almost ten years, he spent only a matter of months in England; the rest of the time he was either at war, on his way to a war or imprisoned. Ranulphus Besace (died *c.* 1243) was the king's physician during the crusade and was probably quite young for the job, to judge from his likely date of death. Meanwhile in London and Normandy, John de Bridport served as the royal doctor.[1]

Neither battle against the powers of Islam, nor the dangers of disease or shipwreck, nor long-term imprisonment in Germany seem to have done the Lionheart any harm, but it all damaged his financial state. Eager to refill his coffers, when he learned that a great treasure of some kind had been found by the lord of Chalûs Castle in Richard's territory of the Limousan in northern France, he was determined to take his share. However, the lord had no intention of sharing and Richard had to resort to besieging Chalûs. During the siege, he was hit in the shoulder by a crossbow bolt, shot from the castle battlements. At the time he thought it quite a minor wound, but twelve days later he died of it. The St Alban's chronicler, Matthew Paris, described the event in some detail:

On March 25th, he [the king] was wounded by a shaft from Peter Basil, poisoned, as was said, but he made light of the injury. Twelve days later, he took the Castle by a furious onslaught. Now the wounds he had received there being badly tended in the meanwhile and beginning to swell, a kind of blackness mingled with the swelling, discolouring the region of the wound on every side; this began to give the king intense pain. The swelling suddenly coming to his heart on April 6th, a day agreed to Mars, the man devoted to martial deeds, breathed his last at the aforesaid Castle.[2]

Matthew Paris seemed to think that his surgeons were to blame for the 'badly tended' wound. Sadly for the king, they may not have read the latest book on surgery by Rogerius, also known as Rogerius Salernitanus or Roger Frugard, from the medical school at Salerno, in Italy. His book entitled *Practica Chirurgiae* (*The Practice of Surgery*) was possibly written around 1180 (sometimes dated earlier to 1170, sometimes later, to 1230). Roger's work is clearly written, brief and practical, arranged anatomically with a suggested treatment for each affliction. He recommended a dressing of egg white (albumen) for wounds of the neck, which may have helped in King Richard's case because it would have sealed the wound. Roger Frugard also discussed arrow wounds to the face with this sensible advice:

If the metal tip is detached, learn from the patient just how he was wounded: in what position he was when he was struck, from above or below, from the front or the side? Then insert a probe into the wound of entry and try to determine the path created by the arrowhead, to find it and to remove it. If you cannot do that without harm to the patient, leave it alone. Many people have lived well ... with metal in them.[3]

Apparently, surgeons at the time of the Napoleonic Wars used the same basic method to find 'missing' musket balls, which was to instruct the patient to 'get into the position you were when hit and say where the shot came from'. Roger's caution about leaving things where they were – if trying to extract them was likely to make matters worse – would probably have been approved too. This seems to have been the case with David II, King of Scots, at the Battle of Neville's Cross in 1346. His face was pierced by two English arrows before he was captured. Taken as a prisoner to York, he was treated by two local barber-surgeons, William of Bolton and Henry de Kilvington. One arrowhead was successfully removed but the other proved too difficult and was left in place. Years later, sometime between 1363 and 1370, David visited the shrine of St Monan in Fife and, as he knelt to pray – so the story goes – the arrowhead emerged from his face and he was miraculously healed.[4]

Returning to Richard the Lionheart, on 1 March 2013 it was reported that, in a new study, scientists had begun to unravel a mystery about the king. When he died, they didn't bury his whole body in a grave or tomb. A man so important, who had ruled not only England but a huge area of France as well, was expected to have his remains spread around, shared between significant towns and cities across his dominions. His body was eviscerated and embalmed; his corpse was entombed at Fontevrault Abbey near Chinon, in Anjou, where his father already lay and his mother, the famous Eleanor of Aquitaine, would join him in 1204, but his heart was placed in a casket to be kept in Rouen Cathedral, in the capital city of his duchy of Normandy. The heart was rediscovered in 1838, inside a lead box, during excavations in the cathedral. A Latin inscription on the lid of the box read, 'Here is the heart of Richard, King of England.' Inside, the heart was no longer recognisable as a human organ – just a pile of brownish powder and a few scraps of the cloth in which it must have been wrapped.

At the time of his death, as Matthew Paris noted above, there were rumours that the crossbow bolt had been tipped with poison and it was hoped that modern science might be able to confirm the presence in Richard's bloodstream of either an infection or a toxic substance which caused his death at the age of just forty-two. Philippe Charlier, a leading forensic expert, and his team were to examine a minute sample of the king's heart material for analysis after 812 years. Monsieur Charlier said that chemical tests on just one or two milligrams of the remains – less than 1 per cent – would be enough to provide conclusive results within three months.[5]

The French scientists who carried out the tests found no traces of poison. The outcome was far more mundane. It seemed most likely that the king died of gangrene when the wound became infected. However, traces of other foreign elements were found, including mercury, which scientists believe would have been used in the embalming process to aid the preservation of the heart. Traces of wood tar and frankincense were also found, along with various fragrant substances which were also probably part of the embalming process.[6] Embalming would have been necessary in Richard's case for practical reasons because it was a long journey from the site of his death in Chalûs to his heart's burial place in Rouen (a distance of about 330 miles). Some historians have speculated that the biblical spices, like frankincense, might have been added to the embalming fluid to hasten Richard's ascent into heaven. Records from the thirteenth century suggest the Church believed his soul sat in purgatory for thirty-three years to purify him of his sins. Mark Ormrod, Professor of History from the University of York, said,

That consciousness of using very high-quality herbs and spices and other materials that are much sought after and rare does add to that sense of it being Christ-like in its quality. Medieval kings were thought to represent the divine on Earth – they were set apart from other lay people and regarded as special and different. So that treatment of the heart strikes me as being absolutely credible.

However efficiently the experts of the time were able to preserve his heart after death, the knowledge of his surgeons hadn't been enough to save Richard the Lionheart's life. But that was in 1199;

by 1403 the skills and techniques of battlefield surgeons had moved on, such that another royal patient fared far better.

Prince Hal – The Battle of Shrewsbury

Henry, Prince of Wales – Shakespeare's 'Prince Hal' and later King Henry V – was aged only sixteen (he had been born at Monmouth on 16 September 1386) when he fought at the Battle of Shrewsbury on 21 July 1403. Young Henry lay injured with a bodkin arrow embedded in his face. It had entered his cheek and the tip was deep into the flesh beside his nose. The shaft was removed, leaving 'the head thereof ... still in the hinder part of the bone of the head [to] the measure of vj (six) inches'.[7] After 'dyverse and wyse lechys' had tried to remove the arrowhead, the surgeon, John Bradmore, used 'tents' – small probes to keep the wound open and enlarge it slightly. These 'tents' were twigs of old elder pith, wrapped with fine linen and dipped in rose honey. Meanwhile, Bradmore directed a blacksmith to make a special pair of fine 'tongs', small, smooth and concave.[8] There was no time or way to test the instrument in advance. Closed, the point of the tongs was inserted into the wound cavity until Bradmore 'imagined' – there were no X-rays, of course – it had entered the hollow part of the arrowhead that had previously held the shaft. Then he used the ingenious screw mechanism to open out the jaws of the tongs until they fitted snugly within the arrowhead and he was able to withdraw the tongs, still gripping the arrowhead, and so removed it. The procedure was completely successful, but there was still the problem of possible infection. Bradmore washed the wound with wine and cleansed it with an ointment containing honey as an antiseptic. The treatment continued for a week and 'afterward the place was helyd' (healed). Bradmore recorded all the details of the operation and follow-up treatment in his book *Philomena*.[9]

Today, we understand that honey draws fluid from the wound,

bringing the bacteria with it. It is also acidic and so discourages bacterial growth. Honey has been used in this way for 4,000 years, but its efficacy is only just being tested scientifically in clinical trials which are proving successful, particularly in healing persistent leg ulcers in the elderly.

As for Prince Hal, he must have been scarred for life and no doubt that is why his portrait as King Henry V is in profile, unlike the three-quarter poses of most other English monarchs. Yet here is another mystery. The surgeon Thomas Morstede, who may have been an eyewitness to the event, also wrote about it in his *Fair Book of Surgery*.[10] He describes the prince's injury and Bradmore's operation as being on 'the lefte syd' of his face, but the left profile is what we see in the king's portrait. Could it be that Morstede didn't know his right from his left? I think one possible explanation is that when looking at the patient from the front, face-on, to perform the procedure, the wound was to the surgeon's left (i.e. the patient's right cheek). Morstede's book contains diagrams and instructions on the making of surgical instruments, including Bradmore's tongs. Sometimes, the contracts drawn up between the king and his medical team on the eve of war specified that they bring not only their instruments, but the equipment needed for making new ones, as required. So it seems that surgeons could turn their hands to the skills of the smithy, although the work must have been more like that of the goldsmith, rather than the blacksmith, but we know that Bradmore did employ a blacksmith to make those special tongs in a hurry.

A Bloody Day – The Battle of Towton

On Palm Sunday, 29 March 1461, the little village of Towton in northern England, between York and Leeds, witnessed what is believed to have been the bloodiest day in English history. Many people have never heard of it and even those who have are forced to look hard to spot the small roadside cross that marks the site of the bloodiest battle ever fought in England. The clash was a turning point in the Wars of the Roses, the dynastic struggle between the rival houses of Lancaster and York. Other quarrels, skullduggery, skirmishes and lesser battles had preceded it, but at Towton the order was issued on both sides that no quarter was to be given. It would be a brutal fight to the death. The weather took a hand as well. A fierce snowstorm blew in the face of the Lancastrian army, blinding the archers and hampering their commanders as they tried to make out what was going on. The result was a crushing victory for the Yorkists and England found herself with a new young king, Edward IV.

In a letter sent nine days after the battle, George Neville, the Chancellor of England, wrote that 28,000 men died that day, a figure that agrees with a letter sent by Edward to his mother. England's total population was probably less than three million and George Goodwin (who wrote a book on Towton to coincide with the battle's 550th anniversary in 2011) reckons as many as 75,000 men, perhaps 10 per cent of the country's fighting-age population, took the field that day.[11]

Lacking a standing army, the royal claimants on both sides called on their allies among the nobility by issuing 'commissions of array' to officers in the shires to raise men. Great lords had followings known as 'affinities' comprised of people on formal retainers (contracts), as well as others with lesser obligations. These soldiers, together with foreign mercenaries in either camp, were the more experienced and better-equipped warriors of the day. Fighting at their side were men from lower down the social scale, who were required by law to practise archery every Sunday after church on the village green. They were not so well trained otherwise, and were unlikely to be able to afford much in the way of protective clothing, except perhaps a helmet and/or buckler. A buckler was a small shield, about the size of a dinner plate, with which to ward off blows.

In the summer of 1996, builders working at Towton Hall, about a mile away from the main battlefield, discovered a mass grave. Archaeologists from the University of Bradford took charge of an excavation of nearly fifty individuals, twenty-eight of whom were complete skeletons. (Further bodies have since been recovered from beneath the dining room at Towton Hall.) The skeletons had clearly been the victims of violence and frenzied attack, many of the injuries being inflicted on their heads. Both the site of their burial and the subsequent carbon dating linked them conclusively to the Battle of Towton. It is the only mass grave of known medieval battle victims to have been found in England. They had been stripped before being thrown into the pit.

Under the supervision of Tim Sutherland – an archaeologist who has been researching the battlefield ever since – the skeletons were carefully recorded, numbered in sequence and their positions mapped in the grave before removal, so that they could be put back together again in the laboratory. From forensic bone analysis it was discovered that all the skeletons were male, with their age at death ranging from sixteen to fifty. Many showed uneven development of their upper limbs, suggesting they were archers. Of all the skeletons, number sixteen – now officially known as 'Towton 16' – proved a significant find. He was strong, quite tall, sturdily built and in his late forties.[12] His head injuries included those inflicted by blades, blunt force trauma caused by heavy blows and a puncture wound, most likely from the spike of a poleaxe, which would have entered the brain. Many of these wounds could have been the fatal one with more inflicted after death, but what is intriguing about Towton 16 is that he had fought in battle before and been seriously wounded, but recovered.

Towton 16 had previously suffered a blade injury to his jaw on the left side of his face. The lesion in the mandibular corpus (jaw bone) is 6.5 centimetres long, where the blade slashed deep enough to damage the bone, so the flesh wound itself would have been longer still. He had lost part of his molar too.[13] This awful injury would have needed surgery at its most skilful level. Part of the bone had been sheared off and the surgeon removed this. All around the injury there are signs that it healed well with no indication that it became infected, leaving Towton 16 fit and well enough to fight another day – when his luck finally ran out. Nevertheless, his recovery is an excellent testimony to the capabilities of the medieval battlefield surgeon.

Would the patient have been conscious and suffering agonies during the procedure to repair his face? Not necessarily. There was the possibility of using an anaesthetic such as 'dwale', as we saw in chapter 3, although it was a risky business. Modern historical films and dramas like to show the wounded being plied with alcohol of some kind before the arrow, musket ball or bullet is removed or the damaged limb amputated, to lessen their pain. However, a good surgeon would have known that alcohol thins the blood, making it slower to coagulate – not a good thing during surgery. The medieval surgeon certainly washed wounds with wine, using it as an antiseptic to cleanse the site of the injury, but to operate on a drunken patient wasn't a wise choice.

After another of Edward IV's victories, this time at the Battle of Barnet in April 1471, Sir John Paston wrote a letter home to his mother, Margaret Paston, in Norfolk. Sir John had fought on the losing side and he tells his mother of the casualties, including his younger brother (also named John). He assures her,

> The two Johns were fortunate; many other Lancastrians, some of exalted rank, died either during the battle or in their flight from the field. It wasn't such a bloody fight as Towton, ten years before, but Richard Neville, Earl of Warwick, and his brother John, Marquis Montague, were both slain.[14]

A Campaign to France
In the summer of 1475 Edward IV was going to war again, but this time it was to be against the French and the event was thoroughly

planned in advance. At the beginning of June, a long document was in the process of being drawn up. Called an indenture, it had the names of all those of any importance who enlisted to serve the king on his French campaign, going 'with our said lord [Edward IV] in thys his Journey towardes the parties of bey yond the See', from the royal dukes of Clarence and Gloucester, each with their own small army, to William Ward, who was bringing thirty labourers to the expedition.[15] In the middle of the indenture is a list of the medical team who would accompany the army and there we find some names already familiar to us.

Magister Jacobus Frise (also known as James or Jacques) heads the medical men as physician to the king; he is to receive 2s per day. Frise is followed by William Hobbys as physician and surgeon – he who disgraced himself with the French prostitutes – but in his dual role he is to be paid the generous sum of 10s 3d per day. It may be that Hobbys had to supply equipment as well out of his pay: instruments, bandages, medications, stretchers and beds for the wounded, perhaps the horses and wagons to carry it all. After Hobbys come seven other surgeons, all to receive wages of 12d per day, among them Richard Esty and Richard Chamber, along with five assistant surgeons to be paid 6d per day, including John Staveley (written in error as 'Stanley' by a later copyist), Hobbys's son-in-law. A little later in the document, for some reason separate from the rest of the medical team, is William Hattecliffe, also hired for the campaign at 2s per day.

Those who hadn't done so already were required to draw up their wills before embarking on the dangers of a campaign. Richard Esty drew up his will on 2 June 1475, referring to himself as a 'yoman Surgen for the body of our said souverain lord'. As it turned out, Edward's 'second Agincourt', as he called it, came to nothing. The king signed a treaty with Louis XI of France instead and none of his surgeons had to wield their scalpels in anger. However, the French plied the English soldiers with free wine, so the medical team may have been called upon to treat a few sore heads and patch up the kind of injuries that result from drunken brawls.

Along with their equipment, the surgeons may well have had 'Wound Men' diagrams. These very graphic and often full-colour images laid out the various wounds that a person might suffer in battle or in accidents, often with surrounding or accompanying text stating treatments for the various injuries. From a cudgel to the head to a caltrop in the foot, the wound man had every conceivable battle injury. Later versions included such weaponry innovations as cutlasses and pistol shot, in addition to the usual cannonball and sword damage. Some historians say these diagrams were to assist the surgeon in an emergency procedure, but I'm more inclined to agree with those who see them as advertisements for display in a surgeon's front window at home, or on a pole outside the medical tent in the field, so everyone could see where to take the wounded. The earliest known wound man in a printed book is found in Johannes de Ketham's *Fasciculus Medicinae*, made in Venice in 1492, but they remained popular in surgical texts throughout the sixteenth century and even into the seventeenth century. Another gory example is in Hans von Gersdorff's *Fieldbook of Wound Surgery*, published in Strasbourg in 1519.

A Most Unfortunate King – Richard III

One battlefield casualty who was completely beyond any surgeon's help was King Richard III after the Battle of Bosworth on 22 August 1485. On 4 September 2012, archaeologists unearthed a skeleton from beneath a car park on what had once been the site of the church of the Greyfriars in Leicester, England. Analysis of the remains, DNA evidence and archaeological evidence from the burial site revealed that the skeleton was that of Richard III, the last English monarch to die on the battlefield. Forensic experts from many fields analysed the skeleton in great detail, using the latest technologies. The bones were those of an adult man with a gracile (slim-boned) build and severe scoliosis of the thoracic spine, with an age-range estimation of thirty to thirty-four years. These findings are consistent with what is known of Richard from contemporary sources: he was thirty-two years old at the time of the battle in 1485, of a slender build with a raised right shoulder.[16]

Richard had suffered at least eleven peri-mortem injuries – that is injuries inflicted around the time of death, which, therefore, show no sign that the healing process had begun – nine of them to the skull. These wouldn't include any number of soft-tissue wounds which left no trace on the bones. All the injuries were consistent with the types of weapons from the late medieval period and the head injuries fit with some near-contemporary accounts of the battle. These sources suggest that Richard abandoned his horse after it foundered in marshy ground and he was killed while fighting his enemies on foot. The injuries would indicate either a sustained attack or an attack by several assailants. The number and severity of the head wounds imply that Richard had either lost his helmet, or it had been removed, perhaps by force, before the injuries to the skull were sustained.[17]

The fact that there seem to be no defensive wounds to the arms and hands means he was still wearing the rest of his armour, but without his helmet, when he died. The most likely fatal injuries were the two to the inferior cranium (base of the skull). One was a penetrating injury from the left side, suggesting that the tip of an edged weapon had pierced through the bone and the brain, as far as the inner surface of the skull opposite the point of entry – a distance of 10.5 centimetres. This wound could have been caused by either a sword tip or perhaps the spike of a halberd. The injuries are consistent with the body having been in a prone position or on its knees with the head pointing downwards.[18]

Three wounds to the face could have been inflicted after death, but they were fairly minor compared to some of the terrible facial injuries from the Battle of Towton, twenty-four years earlier. Historians think that the face was left relatively undamaged because the king's corpse had to be recognisable when it was put on display in Leicester,[19] after the battle, to ensure that there was no doubt that Richard III was dead.

The skeleton had also suffered another serious injury, caused by a fine-bladed weapon (not a staff weapon but more probably a sword) that penetrated the right buttock and went through the right side of the pelvic cavity, in front of the pelvic bones. In life, this injury could have caused damage to the internal organs including the bowel and could have caused substantial, life-threatening bleeding. In battle, Richard's pelvic area would have been protected by either plate or mail armour, or a combination of the two, and beneath those could have been a short mail skirt or a pair of short mail breeches. Therefore, it is most probable that this injury was inflicted after Richard's armour had been removed. Contemporary accounts of the battle describe his body as being slung over the back of a horse and suffering insults and the angle of the injury is consistent with this.[20]

As I've mentioned above, Richard's skeleton, even in its burial pit, was seen to have a severe curvature of the spine; he suffered from scoliosis. This raises some interesting medical questions. Was he born with this problem; could the medicine of the day have helped him in any way and did the curvature affect his everyday life? Would he have been disabled? Experts have determined that Richard wasn't born with scoliosis, but that it developed during the last few years of growth. Known as 'adolescent onset idiopathic scoliosis', the curvature probably began after he was ten years old. The medicine of the time could have done nothing to prevent the curvature increasing – even today, only major surgery can make any difference and is not without risk. Bracing can help in less severe cases of about forty degrees, but is unlikely to have been much use to Richard.

Even so, his physical disfigurement was probably not too noticeable when he was clothed because the curvature was well balanced. His body would have been relatively short in comparison to the length of his limbs and his right shoulder a little higher than the left. However, a good tailor and custom-made armour could have disguised this. At the time of the analysis of Richard's spine, experts suggested his curvature of seventy to ninety degrees would not have impaired his ability to exercise because of a reduced lung capacity. Neither was there any evidence that Richard would have walked with a limp because the leg bones are symmetrical and well formed.[21] He certainly wasn't the hunchback of Tudor propaganda.

Just how mobile and physically able Richard could have been was made apparent during a TV programme, *Richard III: The New Evidence*, screened on Channel 4 on 17 August 2014. A body double for Richard – twenty-seven-year-old Dominic Smee – who has a virtually identical degree of scoliosis to the king, demonstrated what was possible. Without a shirt, his scoliosis was obvious, but clothed it appeared no more than an unevenness in the shoulders. Tobias Capwell, the Curator of Arms and Armour at the Wallace Collection, an expert on fifteenth-century armour and an experienced international jouster himself, showed how a tailor-made suit of armour could be constructed to fit perfectly, the discrepancies only apparent to an intimate observer.

Dominic carried out various exercise routines – some while wearing the armour – and was found to be no less capable than any other man of his age, his lung capacity being within the norm. He was able to bend and twist far more than CT scans had suggested would be the case, so it seems the same may well have been true for Richard. Dominic had never ridden a horse before, but learned how to ride for the experiment. Apparently, he practised by riding his bike in full armour, finding it hampered him hardly at all; the knee joints were flexible enough for pedalling. Surprisingly, on horseback, the medieval bucket-type saddle which Richard would have used proved far more supportive and comfortable for Dominic than a modern one, bracing his back. To prove the point, Dominic rode, fully armoured and armed with a lance, in a joust. He was very successful and demonstrated that Richard was in no way disabled by the scoliosis and would have been the formidable warrior he was described as being, even by his enemies.

The medieval battlefield surgeons would have learned a great deal from their hands-on experience in the field. Just as Galen had learned his anatomy – not always correctly – from dealing with wounded gladiators, centuries before, and practised various methods of cleansing, suturing and aftercare of their injuries before writing it all down, medieval surgeons did much the same. In the next chapter, we will look at how they recorded and passed on their knowledge to next generation.

10

PASSING ON IDEAS

Medicine is a science from which one learns the conditions
    and states
of the human body with regard to health and the absence of
    health ...
the aim being to guard health when it exists and restore it
    when it is lost.

                    Ibn Sina's *Al-Qanum fi al-Tibb, c.* 1025

Physicians studied at university, relying on the ancient texts written
by classical authors, men like Hippocrates, Galen, Aristotle and
Soranus, so it would be hardly surprising if progress in this field
of medicine advanced little from the time of the Romans to the
European Renaissance of the fifteenth, sixteenth and seventeenth
centuries. However, Arab scholars – responsible for rescuing
many ancient Greek texts by translating them into Arabic –
were not reluctant to add their own ideas to the pool of medical
knowledge, among them the Persian Al-Rhazi (*c.* 866–925) and
Ibn Sina (*c.* 980–1037) from Uzbekistan. Their works were later
translated into Latin for western scholars, along with the Greek
writings which were then 'rediscovered' in the twelfth-century
mini-renaissance in Europe.[1]

Gilbertus Anglicus (c. 1180–c. 1250)

Among the Englishmen to benefit from this new-found learning was Gilbertus Anglicus. Gilbert was educated in England as a boy before travelling to Italy, to study at Europe's first and foremost school of medicine at Salerno. His tutor may well have been the renowned physician and surgeon Roger of Parma, because Gilbert quotes Roger extensively in his books. Gilbert returned to England for a few years, to serve the Archbishop of Canterbury, Hubert Walter, but left England again after the archbishop's death in 1205. Known abroad as 'Gilbert the Englishman', he spent the rest of his life on the Continent.

Gilbert compiled a medical encyclopaedia, the *Compendium of Medicine*, written in Latin as the *Compendium Medicinae*, most probably sometime between 1230 and 1250. This was an attempt to bring together all that was best practice in medicine and surgery at the time. The work filled seven books, but Gilbert admitted that much of the material came from the Greeks, like Hippocrates and Galen, from the Arab physicians, Al-Rhazi (Latinised to 'Rhazes') and Ibn Sina (Latinised to 'Avicenna') and their fellows, as well as from Roger of Palma and other masters at Salerno. Well known as a physician across Europe during his lifetime, Gilbert's fame lasted for centuries after his death. His *Compendium* was first produced as a printed edition in 1510 and was reprinted as late as 1608. He even gets a mention in the prologue of Geoffrey Chaucer's *Canterbury Tales*, listed with the greatest medical writers known to Chaucer's physician:

> Wel knew he th'olde Esculapius
> And Deyscorides, and eek Rufus,
> Old Ypocras, Haly and Galien;
> Serapion, Razis and Avycen,
> Averrois, Damascien and Constantyn,
> Bernard and Gatesden and Gilbertyn.[2]

Gilbert's *Compendium Medicinae* was translated into Middle English in the early fifteenth century, making it possible for those who had little knowledge of Latin to read it. Now with a much wider audience – even though books always remained expensive – the chapters on gynaecology and obstetrics were expanded with some new material to become a separate book, known as *The Sickness of Women*. It must have sold well because it was soon rivalling the works of Trotula as the go-to source of information on women's health.[3]

Although he had been a physician, having studied under Roger of Parma – considered a master of physic and surgery – Gilbert had not ignored the surgical aspects of medicine in his encyclopaedia. He also included a selection of apothecaries' remedies; it would have been incomplete otherwise. This is a prescription for the treatment of earache, taken from the Middle English translation of Gilbert's compendium, but versions of the same remedy are found elsewhere in other books in Latin, English and even Dutch:

> Take the bowes of green asshes and ley on the fyer and take of the water that commeth at the endes of hem the quantite of a sponeful and halfe, and put thereto ii spoonful of oile or of botter and oon spoonful of the juse of synegrene [houseleek, Latin name *Sempervivum tectorum*[4]] and ii spoonful of hony and a spoonful of wommannes mylke that norisseth a man childe. And medle all togedre. Then put a drope or ii in the ere and stoppe [plug] it.[5]

As we saw in the previous chapter, the story of surgery was very different. This was a hands-on craft, learned by experience and, particularly on the battlefield, some great advances were made in techniques for dealing with wounded men, tending their injuries and administering medications. Clearly, there would need to be a culture of sharing newly acquired knowledge among the surgeons; how else could progress be made? We have seen that

John Bradmore wrote a detailed account of the methods he used to extract an arrow head from Prince Hal's face in 1403 and the aftercare involved, in his book, *Philomena*. Then Bradmore's assistant, Thomas Morestede, repeated his master's instructions, with diagrams of his surgical instruments, including the special 'tongs' for extracting the arrow head, in his *Fair Book of Surgery*. Apart from practical demonstrations given to apprentices and assistants, handwritten books, pamphlets and papers, followed by printed matter after the mid-fifteenth century, were the surgeons' means of passing on their knowledge to future generations.

Guy de Chauliac (c. 1295–1368)

The Frenchman Guy de Chauliac was one of the most famous surgeons of the Middle Ages. He was probably born, or at least lived, at Chauliac, a village near the southern border of Auvergne, in northern France, coming from a peasant family. Little is known of his early life and education, except for his occasional references to those times in his writings. Guy wrote about his tutors in Toulouse, so we assume that is where he began to study medicine and surgery. He then went on to the University of Montpellier, where the best medical education was then available, and gained his master of medicine degree. In order to receive his degree, he was required to take minor holy orders which, as we've seen, should have meant he couldn't become a surgeon. However, he went to Bologna to attend the lectures on anatomy given by Nicolò Bertuccio and then to Paris, to continue his studies where the famous surgeon Henri de Mondeville had taught and practised.

Guy soon moved on, further south, to practise surgery in the area of Lyons, for ten years or so. He then moved to Avignon, where he accepted the post of physician to Pope Clement VI, sometime between the Pope's election in 1342 and the plague epidemic at Avignon in 1348. It is thought that 'it was seemingly from books that [Chauliac] learned his surgery ... He may have used the knife when embalming the bodies of dead popes, but he was careful to avoid it on living patients.'[6]

Guy was in Avignon when the plague arrived in the city. Unlike most of his fellow practitioners, he stayed to treat the sick, rather than fleeing for his life, and wrote a detailed report on the epidemic. He wasn't impressed by the way the rest of the medical fraternity deserted the afflicted, but he also realised how little could be done:

> The plague was shameful for the physicians who could give no help at all, especially as, out of fear of infection, they hesitated to visit the sick. Even if they achieved nothing and earned no fees, for all those who caught the plague died, except for a few towards the end of the epidemic who escaped after the buboes had ripened.[7]

Presumably, he was one of those few for he claimed that he too had caught the plague and survived by treating himself. Through close observations, Guy distinguished two forms of the disease, the bubonic and the pneumonic, and as a precaution he advised Pope Clement to keep a fire burning continuously in his chamber and to keep visitors out. He gave this description to the papal court:

> The great death toll began in our case in the month of January [1348], and lasted for the space of seven months. It was of two kinds: the first lasted two months; with continuous fever and spitting of blood; and death occurred within three days. The second lasted for the whole of the remainder of the time, also with continuous fever, and with ulcers and boils in the extremities, principally under the arm-pits and in the groin; and death took place within five days. And [it] was of so great a contagion (especially when there was spitting of blood) that not only through living in the same house but merely through looking, one person caught it from the other.[8]

Guy had seen that the plague could take different forms and explained this to his fellows. The first form described, the pneumonic plague, with one of its symptoms being the 'spitting of blood', was the far more contagious. In 1363, now the first physician to Pope Urban V, he finished bringing together material for his most important work: *Chirurgia magna (Great Surgery)*. It opens with a historical review of medicine as he saw it and included his opinions on other medical sources available to him in the mid-fourteenth century. He thoroughly approved of the texts of Galen which had lately been translated from Greek into Latin, but didn't think much of John of Gaddesden's *Rosa Anglica*. Guy's *Chirurgia magna*, translated into many languages and passed through countless editions, was still one of the most important books on surgery used until the eighteenth century. He died just five years later, in 1368.[9]

Thomas Fayreford (fl. 1400–1450)

Thomas Fayreford was a medical practitioner, working in the West Country, in England, at sometime during the first half of the fifteenth century. We only know of his existence because he put together what he called a 'commonplace book' – a combination of notebook and journal which included a list of cures he had carried out in Oxford in the first decade of the fifteenth century. This book still exists at the British Library as Harley MS 2558, which has been digitised and can be viewed online.[10] It is the only source we have of information for his life and work. He mentions seeing Nicholas Colnet in Oxford, administering a cure, most probably before 1410. Scholars think Thomas may have studied at the university there and collected his information from the libraries.

The book is written mostly in Latin with some Middle English and includes treatises on uroscopy, surgery and alchemy, as well as a section on herbs. These texts he copied from other sources in his own hand, in a style that suggests he wrote them up in his commonplace book a little later, in the second quarter of the century. But the list of cures, entitled 'Cures performed by Thomas Fayreford in different places', giving details of patients' names, occupations and places of residence, the ailments that afflicted them and the treatments given, is unique.[11] In some cases there is a prognostication: *quod omnes disperaverunt de vita eius* (that all despaired of his life).[12] The list has 103 entries – all undated, unfortunately. One patient is noted as living in Fairford, in Gloucestershire, which was probably Thomas's hometown and main place of work, although he travelled around quite a bit in the course of his practice.

We know he worked at Bridgwater in Somerset and Tiverton in Devon, with other patients spread around north-west Devon, from Linton to Barnstaple. Quite how he arranged his visits to such a wide area, we don't know. Not only were his patients well spread across at least three counties, they seem to have come from widely differing social backgrounds as well: from Lady Poynings to the daughter of a humble cook named Geoffrey, from members of the clergy to tradesmen, including a miller and a cellarer. Over half his patients were men, but he treated women and children too, often for minor problems, such as splinters, burns and scalds, to fractured limbs – all in a surgeon's remit. He treated a youngster with an injury to his eye:

There was a boy from Tiverton in Devon about twelve years of age who lost the sight of one eye after a blow to it, so that he could not see at all with the other eye closed. Twice daily I put in the affected eye swallow's blood and daily he drank betony mashed up with ale, and within fifteen days he recovered his sight by the grace of God.[13]

He goes on to note that drinking betony in this form and bathing the eye with rosewater also works. Yet Thomas's field of expertise went further, encroaching on problems usually dealt with by physicians, including treating fevers and gynaecological ailments. The most common female problem seems to have been 'suffocation of the womb' which troubled Lady Poynings and a number of other women. Thomas wasn't one to avoid these intimate, feminine problems, despite other contemporary sources implying that male medieval practitioners kept well away from such womanly complaints. The unfortunate Lady Poynings was also suffering from frenzy, syncope (fainting fits) and quinsy, as well as her gynaecological problem, all at the same time. Thomas, though, says she was cured in three weeks.[14] He also cured Lord Poynings of gout.

Thomas kept a note of the remedies he used in his commonplace book. Some came from books written by the likes of Bernard de Gordon or Gilbertus Anglicus, such as the treatment Thomas administered to an elderly woman from Northover in Somerset. She was afflicted with *cephalargica* (a headache accompanied by nausea) and a painful tremor in her stomach. Her mouth was twisted and her tongue got in the way of her speech – maybe she had suffered a slight stroke. For three weeks he had her gargling, injected her through the nostrils, bled her from beneath the tongue, anointed her head, purged her, gave her Jerusalem pills and dosed her with theriac.[15] Jerusalem pills were a powerful purgative.[16] Other remedies he collected and tested during the course of his work, listed under the headings of the diseases they treated. Some he gleaned from fellow physicians, as well as from his clientele and people whom he met in the course of his work. In a few examples, Thomas says who gave them to him and whether the 'experiment' was successful. Lady Poynings told him of a herbal remedy for *demigreyne* (migraine) and Friar John of London gave him another for the same problem. There is also a recipe for extracting a tooth by means of a frog that Thomas said was his 'privyte', or secret, and which he 'sold' on to another practitioner.[17] He treated John Cloode who suffered headaches, delirium and fever:

One (Cloode) often had headache to the point of delirium. I had his head shaved and with plantain mixed with houseleek and verbena, I washed his head using sharp wine. Then I anointed him with an ointment made of poplar buds, rose and camomile oil mixed up together. Immediately he said that his head was healed, although for a long time he had suffered from hectic fever.[18]

We learn from his book that Thomas was just as likely to use charms as medical treatments and we know other doctors did the same – a perfectly respectable practice at the time. As an example, a charm for treating epilepsy – the 'falling sickness' – is listed alongside a more logical remedy for the same problem:

Write the word of power, *ananzapta*, onto a parchment. This, together with a piece of mistletoe taken from an oak, is for the patient to wear around the neck. The patient must say three masses of the Trinity and eat root of peony daily.[19]

He also used charms with religious connotations, like this one from his commonplace book, which is a 'medicine ffor to stanche blod':

First have the name of the man or woman then go to church and say this charm, and see that you say it only for a man or woman. 'When our lord Jesus Christ was put on the cross then Longinus came there and stabbed him with his spear in the side. Blood and water came out at the wound, and he wiped his eyes.' Then say straight away 'Through the holy virtue that God (gives?) then I conjure thee, blood, that thou do not come out of this Christian man', and name his name twice over, 'Name Name'. 'In the name of the Father and the Son and the Holy Ghost, Amen'. Say this charm three times, nor is it necessary to know where the man or woman is, as long as you know their name.[20]

Historians think that Thomas wrote the book with the purpose of handing on the information and medical 'secrets' to an apprentice,[21] if he had one, or else to his fellow professionals.

Sharing Knowledge and Information

Thomas Fayreford wasn't the only practitioner to write a commonplace book in order to preserve and pass on what he had learned during his years of treating patients. Doctor John Argentine's medical recipes, recorded in Latin in his commonplace book, include the 'experiment' of a Hertfordshire woman who cured a friar of sciatica in 1476, and of Argentine's colleague, William Ordew, who successfully treated a Cambridgeshire rector with a case of 'hectic fever'.[22] This shows a willingness, even among university-trained physicians, to make use of the findings of fellow practitioners, women as well as men, and share their knowledge. A recipe, written in English in 1471, to either prevent or cure the plague was attributed to King Edward IV,[23] showing how important the sharing of medical knowledge was considered to be, even by royalty.

We have heard a little about Thomas Morestede's *Fair Book of Surgery* which seemed to borrow freely from John Bradmore's work, but Morestede went on to cover other items of practical knowledge and expertise, as well as theory, writing in Middle English:

To know the ryght cours how the waynys arteryes cordis or swyth othyr maner thynge be the wyche the surgen schall rather exchew perell in incusyons.

(To know the right course, how the veins, arteries, heart or such other manner [of] things by which the surgeon shall rather eschew peril [avoid danger] in incisions).[24]

Morstede went into detail on how to set broken bones, instructing that care must be taken not to damage ligaments or nerves when articulating the bones – all practical advice. He described and illustrated various surgical instruments, their applications and uses, the formulation of medicines, syrups, poultices and plasters, but was also concerned with the theoretical relationship between surgery and physic: 'Yt may welbe sayd ther for that phesyke ys a universall crafte & surgery but partyculor crafte ther of' (It may well be said therefore that physic is a universal craft and surgery but a particular craft thereof).[25]

He listed the accomplishments that a surgeon ought to have in order to qualify as an 'experte', namely that he should be 'eloquent & lettyrd', have an understanding of the principles of surgery 'in theoryke as in the practyke', to be 'comprehendyd in athonamy [*sic*] ... of mannys body', as well as being pleasant to look at, steady-handed and merciful to poor folk.[26] Morstede's book appears to be quite comprehensive, covering virtually every aspect of surgery.

The sharing of such knowledge and expertise spread far wider than simply from master to apprentice, as shown by the bequests made by many surgeons and barbers, leaving their books to posterity. Richard Esty, a barber-surgeon and yeoman-surgeon to Edward IV, left his seven books of surgery, among other items, to the Fellowship of the Barbers of London in his will of 1475.[27] Thomas Colard, a barber, in 1481, left two books to his son for his lifetime, 'both be of fysyk and surgery' which were to be donated to the library of the hall of Barbers after the son's death and Hugh Herte, barber surgeon, in 1467, left a book of surgery to 'the commonalty of the Art of Surgeons'[28]. 'Guido', the book bequeathed by both John Hobbys (father of William Hobbys) and John Dagvile the younger, may well have been the book *Anathomia*, and was possibly used as a teaching aid by the barber-surgeons as it was well illustrated with anatomical diagrams.

Anathomia was compiled by the Italian Guido de Vigevano around 1340 and had been used to illustrate his anatomy classes by the influential teacher Henri de Mondeville in the fourteenth century.[29] Therefore, there was a long tradition of using 'Guido' for teaching purposes that the barber-surgeons may well have continued.

Guido da Vigevano (*c.* 1280–*c.* 1349) was an Italian physician and engineer, the first to use pictures to illustrate his descriptions, combining medical study with artistic drawings – an idea that was taken further in the Renaissance, as we'll see in chapter 11. In his textbook *Anathomia* there are six images showing for the first time various anatomical structures and the techniques for dissecting them. The head was dissected by the method of trephination, or trepanning (making a hole in the skull) to show the meninges – the three layers of connective tissue that protect the brain and spinal cord – the cerebrum and the spinal cord itself. Guido was the first to illustrate his anatomical descriptions with diagrams to help students to understand the complex structures.[30]

Guido was also an inventor, a forerunner of Leonardo da Vinci, drawing sketches of armoured chariots and siege engines. As physician to the Queen of France, Jeanne de Bourgogne – also known as Joan the Lame – he created a vehicle that moved using a windmill that, via a system of gears similar to those in a mill, turned the wheels.[31] Was this the first car in history?

This evidence shows how freely and openly knowledge and information were shared among medical practitioners. Some practitioners compiled their own medical texts or added to copies of existing manuscripts with the clear implication that they were intended for the use of their fellows, as well as for personal reference. Although some texts, like those of John Argentine, were written in Latin, other authors wrote in the vernacular, like Thomas Morstede. Others, like Thomas Fayreford, mixed both Latin and English, making their information more accessible to a growing literate audience. Writing in Middle English may also have served to make the public, outside the medical fraternity, more aware of the 'professional' attitudes and the expertise of practitioners, as well as encouraging apprentices to the crafts of physic, surgery and, perhaps, even apothecaries, to study the compiled information.

Almost 1,500 years had passed since Galen had 'improved' on the Hippocratic writings, defining the theories of the humours to their most elaborate form, yet his books were still the 'holy writ' of the medical profession. But surely things cannot have remained unchanged for so long; progress must have been made. In the next chapter, we will explore some of the new ideas developing in Tudor medicine and determine whether progress had been made – or not.

II

TUDOR MEDICINE

A good cook is half a physician. The chief physick [medicine] doth come from the kitchen wherefore the physician and the cook must consult together.

Andrew Boorde
Compendyous Regyment or Dyetary of Health, 1542

In this chapter, we will look at some of the changes occurring in medicine in the sixteenth century. We've seen how surgery was slowly developing through practical experiment with the treating of injuries and the handing on of that knowledge from master to apprentice. But what of the university-trained physicians? Had their theoretical knowledge advanced at all? Or were they still relying on Aristotle and Galen, those same old textbooks that had been their source of knowledge since Roman times?

Andrew Boorde (c. 1490–1549)
The Tudor physician Andrew Boorde had been born at Borde Hill near Cuckfield, Sussex, in England, and he wrote of his new ideas, although they don't seem to be very progressive. Boorde was educated at the University of Oxford, taking his vows as a monk

when he was twenty-five, in 1515. He entered the Carthusian order at the London Charterhouse, but just two years later he was accused of being 'conversant with women'.[1] He couldn't put up with the strict regime of the Carthusians, who were against drink and ate no meat, and so he applied to be released from his vows. His request was granted in 1528 and Boorde went abroad to study medicine at as many universities as he could, visiting those of Orléans, Poitiers, Toulouse, Montpellier and Wittenberg. In Rome, he saw 'much abominable vices' and decided to complete his European tour with a pilgrimage to Santiago de Compostela in Spain.[2] His ideas on what constituted a healthy diet show why he couldn't live like a monk:

A lord's dish, good for an Englishman, for it makes him strong and hardy: beef, so be it the beast be young and it must not be cow flesh nor over salted. Veal is good and easily digested; boar's meat is a usual dish in winter for Englishmen.

Ale for an Englishman is a natural drink. Ale must have these properties, it must be fresh and clear, it must not be ropy, nor smoky, nor it must have no weft nor tail ... Beer is made of malt, of hops and water; it is a natural drink for a Dutchman, and now, of late days, it is much used in England to the detriment of many Englishmen ... for it doth make a man fat and doth inflate the belly, as it doth appear by the Dutchmen's faces and bellies.[3]

Boorde returned to England in 1530 and attended Thomas Howard, Duke of Norfolk, when he was sick. The duke must have been pleased with Boorde's work because he asked him to treat the king, Henry VIII. We don't know whether he did or not, but there is no record of any payment made to Boorde from the king's privy purse expenses. In his spare moments, he wrote the first known English travellers' guidebook to Europe.

His so-called new ideas were not always a step forward, as in his healthy lifestyle tips for Englishmen that included no beer or bathing. In his book *Compendyous Regyment or Dyetary of Health*, printed in 1542, he made the far more sensible observation that eating too much shortens a man's life – two meals a day should suffice, except for a labourer who may require three. 'As for carters and ploughmen,' Boorde went on, 'bacon is good for them. Slices of bacon and eggs are very wholesome for such folk.' His dietary instructions explained that

bread should be of wheat alone, not mixed grains, but oatcake is a lordly dish also. Pottage is eaten more often in England than anywhere else in Christendom and it is made by adding oatmeal, herbs and seasoning into boiling meat stock. Or an Englishman might enjoy a nourishing, strength-building frumenty, made by stewing meat and wheat in milk. Otherwise, milk is only good for old men, melancholy men, children and consumptives.

A bustard is nutritious meat and a bittern is not so hard to digest as a heron. Plovers and lapwings are not so nourishing as turtle-doves. Of small birds, the lark is best; thrushes are also good, but not titmouses or wrens, because they eat spiders.[4]

Bustards were then fairly common birds that lived on the Downlands. (There have been recent efforts to reintroduce them.) They are heavy and prefer to run rather than fly and so were easily caught. There was a medieval joke that if you wanted to catch a bustard, you took a net out onto the hillside and, when you caught sight of the bird, you stared at the ground as if at something of great interest. The bustard, being a most inquisitive creature, would come close to see what you were looking at, then you flung the net over him and he was trapped.

Boorde wrote that England had the best fish: sea fish, freshwater fish and all kinds of salted fish. He said sea fish were more wholesome than river fish, which tasted of mud. Since Henry VIII ruled that all Englishmen had to eat fish on Saturdays – this because the fishermen of Grimsby knew not what else to do with the surplus herrings in their nets – as well as Wednesdays and Fridays, as the Church required, Boorde reminded his readers that fish and flesh should not be eaten at the same meal, however much the diners may be tempted. He advised that Englishmen should eat turnips, parsnips, carrots, onions, leeks, garlic and radishes. Mellow red apples were considered very good, but 'beware of green sallettes and rawe fruytes for they wyll make yowr soverayne seke'.

As you can see, very little had changed regarding what was believed to be a medically sound, healthy diet, but concerning drinking water Boorde thought it should never be drunk by itself, but could be used to dilute wine. He was wise enough to realise that 'rain water was best, next came running water, and lastly, well water. Standing water engendered illness, ale being the natural drink for an Englishman'. For those who had drunk too much ale or wine the previous evening, he recommended drinking a dish of milk in the morning.

Sleep was another subject that Boorde dealt with in his *Compendyous Regyment*. Apparently, a healthy man should not sleep by day, but if he must do so,

let him lean and sleep against a cupboard, or else sitting upright in a chair. At night, there must be a fire in the bedchamber to purify the air and consume evil vapours and the windows must be kept closed. Seven hours sleep is enough for a man but he must sleep on his right side with the head high; have a good, thick quilt and let his night-cap be of scarlet. To counteract fear, use merry company, rise in the morning with mirth and remember God. Mirth is one of the chiefest things in physic.

Despite his travels across Europe and his visits to the Continental universities, it seems that this English physician had hardly moved on in his medical knowledge, but elsewhere, others were beginning to break new ground.

In Europe, the Renaissance in art, literature and culture was well underway. New ideas in every field of science and art was being tentatively explored and, whatever the Church, the State or orthodox opinion might do in an effort to prevent it, an inexorable landslide of novel and controversial ways of thinking had begun.

Paracelsus (1493–1541)

At the head of this landslide, Theophrastus Aureolus Bombastus von Hohenheim was born in Switzerland, the son of a physician. Having studied medicine in Italy, he then became a surgeon in the Venetian army. Like Galen and Dioscorides before him, he travelled widely with the military throughout Europe and also journeyed to Egypt, Arabia and even Russia. He wrote of his experiences as an army doctor in his book *Die große Wundarzney*, perhaps the first work on antisepsis. At a time when many doctors believed that infection was a natural part of the healing process, he was an advocate for cleanliness and protection of wounds, as well as the regulation of diet.[5]

Wherever he went, he was interested in the medicine of the people, their folk remedies and knowledge of local plants and geology. He later admitted that he wasn't ashamed of having learned information from 'tramps, butchers and barbers'.[6] Having come by much of his knowledge from these unorthodox sources, he began to realise some of the shortcomings of university-taught medicine and even began to question the classical authorities on the subject.

With his revolutionary thinking, he changed his name to Paracelsus ('equal to Celsus') to show that he regarded himself as a rival to the ancients, men like Galen and Celsus. He discounted Galen's explanations of good health or sickness being the result of whether or not the four bodily humours were in balance. He claimed that the only way to learn medicine was to study nature and, even more controversially, to carry out experiments and observe the results personally. He stated that 'patients are the only books' and called Galen 'a liar and a fake'.[7] This all sounds quite modern but, strangely, he was still back in the dark ages with his belief in fairies, elves and gnomes.

In 1526 he had been appointed to the post of Professor of Medicine at the University of Basel, Switzerland. Having such a poor opinion of the writings of Galen, Hippocrates and others was one thing, but Paracelsus demonstrated his complete rejection of classical medicine, having his students burn the conventional textbooks on a great public bonfire.[8] He disapproved of bloodletting, asking how reducing the amount of blood in the body could possibly be a means of purifying it or removing the harmful components. Having dismissed the theory of the four humours, Paracelsus replaced it with another, no less complicated, 'three principles' theory with the essential elements being sulphur, mercury and salt. He explained this in his *Opus paramirum* in 1530. Sulphur, mercury and salt had been important in medieval alchemy and he demonstrated his theory by burning a piece of wood. The fire was the work of sulphur, the smoke was mercury and the residual ash was salt. It followed, according to his ideas, that these three principles contained the poisons that caused all diseases and, therefore, each disease had three separate cures, depending on whether it was being caused by the poisoning of sulphur, mercury or salt.

At the university, he took the unprecedented step of welcoming the people of Basel to his lectures, as willing to share his knowledge with ordinary folk as to learn from them. In order to stress his lack of respect for the formal methods of teaching, he preferred to wear an alchemist's leather apron rather than an academic gown.

Paracelsus was also an alchemist, carrying out experiments in the manner of a chemist: heating, distilling, reacting and sublimating all kinds of compounds. From this field of his work, he determined that metals were the key elements which made up the universe. They, in turn, were governed by God, whom he saw as the 'great magician' who created Nature.[9] He was the first to use the name 'zink' (for the element zinc) in 1526, because of the sharp-pointed appearance of its crystals after smelting, from the Old German word 'zinke' for pointed. He was especially interested in the illnesses suffered by German miners and workers in the smelting industry. He became a pioneer in the field of industrial diseases and wrote a major work *On the Miners' Sickness and Other Diseases of Miners*, dealing with the occupational hazards of metalworking, their treatment and possible means of prevention.

Although it cannot be proven, Paracelsus may have been the first European doctor to use laudanum as an analgesic. Laudanum is an opium preparation in alcohol, especially effective in easing the pain of battlefield injuries. He may have come across the drug on a visit to Constantinople. Another, more certain, important contribution of his to medicine was the study of the benefits and curative powers of alpine mineral spring waters. His travels brought him to areas of the Alps where such 'taking the waters' therapies were already practised, although not widely known elsewhere at the time. Such treatments would have been thought of as alchemy.

Paracelsus summarised his views on alchemy: 'Many have said of Alchemy, that it is for the making of gold and silver. For me such is not the aim, but to consider only what virtue and power may lie in medicines,'[10] He imagined the human body as a chemical system – rather than a humoral one – which had to be in balance internally, as well as being in harmony with the external environment, in order to have good health. The table below shows how he believed the universe, the known metals and the organs of human body related harmoniously to each other:

Planet	Metal	Organ affected
Sun	Gold	Heart
Moon	Silver	Brain
Jupiter	Tin	Liver
Venus	Copper	Kidneys
Saturn	Lead	Spleen
Mars	Iron	Gall bladder
Mercury	Quicksilver	Lungs

Thinking about the chemistry of the body, rather than the four humours, led Paracelsus to introduce a wide range of new chemical and mineral substances into medicine as possible remedies. As an example, he was the first to use mercury as a treatment for syphilis – the great pox – a lethal medication that, nevertheless, was still being administered in the nineteenth century.

His rule of thumb was that if a poison caused a disease, that same poison might also prove to be the cure, if it was given in the correct dosage and formulation: 'All things are poison and nothing is without poison – only the dose permits something not to be poisonous.' Literally, he was saying that evil could overcome evil, that poisons could have beneficial medical effects. Because everything in the universe was interrelated, beneficial medical substances could be found in all herbs and minerals and any combinations of these. His heretical idea that the universe was a single coherent organism, mankind included, governed by one life-giving entity, God, put him at odds with the Church. Not surprisingly, the university authorities took exception to his lecturing style and his outrageous new ideas and in 1538 he was exiled from Basel.

Paracelsus was undeterred by his rejection. After all, in his own words,

> I am Theophrastus and greater than those to whom you liken me ... I need not don a coat of mail or a buckler against you, for you are not learned or experienced enough to refute even a word of mine ... Let me tell you this: every little hair on my neck knows more than you and all your scribes and my shoe buckles are more learned than your Galen and Avicenna, and my beard has more experience than all your high colleges.[11]

He died in exile in Salzburg, Austria, in 1541, but doubts had been sown about some of the ideas and theories in classical medicine – doubts that would never go away.

Andreas Versalius (1514–64)

With Paracelsus daring to question the ancient authorities, others soon followed his lead and Andreas Versalius, born in Brabant (now in Belgium), was one of the pioneers. He wrote perhaps the most influential of early books on human anatomy, *De humani corporis fabrica* (*On the Fabric of the Human Body*) and is regarded as the founder of the modern science of anatomy. At the age of only twenty-three, he became Professor of Surgery and Anatomy at the University of Padua.

Gradually, since the early 1300s, human dissection was coming to play a small part in medical training. The students at Bologna, in Italy, had been the first to attend human dissections as part of the course and the idea began to spread through Italy, then Spain, then elsewhere, although the English universities lagged behind. Neither the students nor the master physician in charge actually got their hands dirty. The master, seated high in the anatomy theatre, directed a barber-surgeon to carry out the dissection while the students observed. That was the traditional way, but Versalius changed all that.

His interest in learning human anatomy from the body itself, not from an ancient textbook, had begun early on. This is his story of how, as a youngster, he stole the body of a hanged man from a gibbet in Louvain, in Belgium:

> The bones were entirely bare, held together by the ligaments alone ... I climbed the gallows and pulled off the femur from the hip bone ... After I had brought the legs and arms home in secret (leaving the head behind with the trunk of the body), I let myself be locked out of the city in the evening in order to obtain the trunk ... The next day I transported the bones home piecemeal.[12]

As well as teaching at Padua, Versalius also gave lectures at Bologna and Pisa. Previously, as we've seen, anatomy was taught primarily from reading classical texts, mainly Galen, backed up with animal dissections. No attempt had been made to actually check on the things Galen said about the human form; his word was unquestionable. However, Vesalius had other ideas about how the subject should be taught. He conducted dissections personally, seeing them as the best and primary teaching aid, wielding the scalpel himself and having the students perform dissections to see for themselves exactly how the human body looked internally. Although he had begun by examining the bone structure of the hanged man, he also dissected the musculature, major organs, the nervous system and the arterio-venous system. He taught that hands-on direct observation was the only reliable resource of anatomical information.

Teaching in this way was a complete break with medieval practice, but Versalius' new methods of instruction didn't end there. The printing press was now operating across Europe and

Versalius made full use of the latest technology to spread his knowledge of human anatomy. His book *De humani corporis fabrica* was first printed and published in 1543 with twenty-three full-page anatomical illustrations and 180 smaller diagrams to aid the reader. In Padua, Versalius had got to know a few artists who dissected bodies to improve the realism of their painted figures, among them one of his fellow countrymen, Jan Stephan van Calcar. Calcar was an apprentice to the master artist Titian.[13] Calcar did some of the drawings for Versalius' book, which was printed in Basle, Switzerland, by Johannes Oporinus, a man known for his skill and care in producing the finest woodcuts – illustrations that made *De humani corporis* unique among medical textbooks.[14]

In carrying out his own dissections, Versalius was able to discover that Galen had been mistaken in some cases in applying what he'd seen in monkeys and pigs to human anatomy. This is what Versalius wrote after studying the human jaw:

> The jaw of most animals is formed of two bones joined together at the apex of the chin where the lower jaw ends in a point. In man, however, the lower jaw is formed of a single bone ... Galen and most of the skilled dissectors after the time of Hippocrates asserted that the jaw is not a single bone. However this may be, so far no human jaw has come to my attention constructed of two bones.

Galen had also believed that, in the heart, the blood leaked across from one side of the organ to the other through holes in the septum (the membrane down the centre of the heart), although these were too small to be seen. Versalius, and later the Englishman William Harvey (1578–1657), proved why the holes were invisible – they aren't there! Galen had no idea that the two sides of the heart were entirely separate: one half receiving the blood, via the veins, from the rest of the body and pumping it to the lungs to exchange carbon dioxide for oxygen; the other half receiving the now oxygenated blood from the lungs and pumping it back round the body via the arteries. The heart has these two distinct circulatory systems, but Galen had no idea that blood circulated at all. Versalius spotted the evidence and William Harvey would explain how it worked in a lecture in 1616 and publish his findings in his book *De motu cordis* (*The Motions of the Heart*). It was Harvey who developed the idea of the blood circulating in one direction only – Galen had thought that it ebbed and flowed like the sea. Harvey's old professor of Anatomy at the University of Padua in Italy, Hieronymous Fabricius (*c.* 1533–1619), had noticed the little flaps of tissue in the veins that served as non-return valves, preventing any backflow of blood.[15] Harvey thought this discovery through to its ultimate conclusion and is credited with revealing the circulation of the blood. English medicine was beginning to move on, at last.

Leonardo da Vinci (1452–1519)

It may seem odd to include a man famous for his art in a book about medicine, but decades before Versalius was compiling the beautiful anatomical drawings for his *De humani corporis fabrica*, Leonardo was making detailed sketches of the human form, both internally and externally, in order that the depictions of people in his art should be perfectly lifelike. His interest seems to have begun at the beginning of his career, during his apprenticeship, and by the 1490s it had become an important part of his research. Studying the structure of the human body, Leonardo tried to understand how it functioned. For twenty years, he did practical work in dissecting in Milan and then at hospitals in Florence, Rome and Pavia.

In 1506, Leonardo's acquaintance with a young professor of anatomy, Marcantonio della Torre, led the artist to undertake many first-hand human dissections; he reckoned he had dissected thirty corpses in his lifetime.[16] Four years later the expertise he gained with the help of della Torre would prove useful in his studies of embryology. The series of drawings done between 1510 and 1512 were drawn with black and red chalk with some pen-and-ink wash on paper. These groundbreaking illustrations correctly depict the human foetus in its proper position within the womb. Leonardo was also the first to expertly depict the uterine artery and the vascular system of the cervix and vagina, drawing the uterus with only one chamber. This contradicted the ancient theory that the uterus was made up of many chambers which, so it was believed, divided foetuses into separate compartments in the case of twins.

One of the most famous of his drawings is that of an unborn baby in the womb, correctly attached by the umbilical cord, yet the drawing has one obvious mistake – there are projections, called cotyledons, within the wall of the womb which are found in ungulates, in a cow's or sheep's uterus, but not in humans.[17]

Despite his error, these drawings were all so different from the medieval diagrams of babies in the womb. In these earlier illustrations the uterus is shown like an inverted flask, narrow-necked and bulbous, in which the foetus is a miniature adult with adult proportions: small head and long limbs relative to the size of the trunk. The foetus floats freely in the womb, unattached in any way. This is yet another mystery: how medieval doctors could imagine that the unborn foetus in the womb looked so unlike a newborn baby in its proportions.[18]

Apart from his drawings of the female anatomy, Leonardo's sketches reveal an in-depth knowledge of how the human body functioned, much of it still in tune with our understanding today. Only in the twentieth century did modern anatomists study the muscles and tendons of the finger in the same detail as Leonardo. He was the first to draw the human spine with the correct curvature and came so close to understanding how blood moved through the body, a mystery that was finally solved by William Harvey over a century later,[19] as we shall see in chapter 12.

The Royal College of Physicians

In the first quarter of the sixteenth century, the physicians of London decided it was time they had their own authority to regulate the practice of medicine in England. The surgeons and apothecaries had their own companies to oversee the granting of licences and permission to practise and the physicians felt they were missing out. The leading physicians also wanted the power to grant licences to those qualified in medicine and the authority to punish untrained practitioners and those involved in malpractice of various kinds: practising while unqualified, negligent or outright charlatans. In 1518, a small group of physicians petitioned King Henry VIII, requesting permission to establish a college of physicians.[20] The king agreed and granted them a royal charter founding the College of Physicians of London, the oldest medical college in England. The charter stated that the college was authorised to 'curb the audacity of those wicked men who shall profess medicine more for the sake of their avarice than from the assurance of any good conscience, whereby many inconveniences may ensue to the rude and credulous populace'.[21]

At first the college only had jurisdiction in London, but in 1523 an Act of Parliament extended their licensing powers to the whole of England. In the original charter, the new authority was called the College of Physicians or the King's College of Physicians. It only gradually became known as the 'Royal College of Physicians of London' during the seventeenth century.

Among those who had petitioned the king, the most influential was the royal physician Thomas Linacre (*c.* 1460–1524), who had travelled throughout Europe and seen the way medicine was regulated in other cities. Linacre was born near Chesterfield, in Derbyshire, but went to school at Canterbury Cathedral School before studying at All Souls College, Oxford, and then at the University of Padua. He had been both the physician and tutor to Prince Arthur – Henry VIII's late elder brother – and became

Henry's own physician in 1509. Among his other duties at court, Linacre was also Princess Mary Tudor's Latin teacher and Cardinal Wolsey was one of his many affluent patients. Linacre was appointed as the first president of the College of Physicians and the members held their meetings at his house in Knightrider Street, near St Paul's Cathedral, in London.

As president, Linacre wanted the college to be an academic body for physicians, not a kind of trade guild such as those that regulated the surgeons and apothecaries. Physicians were regarded as the educated elite of the medical world, needing to have a university degree in order to gain a licence. Candidates wanting to become fellows of the college had to sit an oral examination, to demonstrate their classical knowledge as well as their medical expertise.

From the very beginning, the College of Physicians was in conflict with the other medical governing bodies in London. The struggle to control the licensing system in the capital led to bitter rivalry between the college and the Company of Barber-Surgeons in particular. With the elitist physicians snubbing the surgeons at every opportunity, this was a very different attitude from that of 1423, when the two groups had attempted to cooperate in the conjoined College of Physicians and Surgeons. However, with less than sixty fellows at any one time during the sixteenth century, and never more than 100 licentiates, the far more numerous surgeons and apothecaries felt at liberty to treat the rapidly expanding population of London without reference to the physicians, despite the latter's best efforts to enforce their regulations and licensing procedure. The college's threat of fines and imposed restrictions didn't carry much weight either.

The college was partly to blame for the situation. It didn't take the lead in the broader medical profession, preferring to sit back and wait on events and so was seen as a very conservative establishment. It refused to allow anyone to join the fellowship who had not been to either Oxford or Cambridge universities, a regulation that continued until 1835. Of course, women were completely excluded until 1909, when a bylaw was passed allowing them to take the entry examinations.

John Caius (1510–73)

One of Linacre's successors as president of the Royal College of Physicians of London was John Caius. Caius was born in Norwich, Norfolk, in 1510. He became a student at what was then Gonville Hall, Cambridge, where he studied divinity. After graduating in 1533, he went to Padua to study medicine under Andreas Vesalius, gaining his degree in physic in 1541. In 1543, he visited other parts of Italy, Germany and France before returning to England. He was a physician in London in 1547 and was admitted as a fellow of the College of Physicians (he would go on to become its president nine times). In 1557, being the royal physician to Mary Tudor, he was wealthy enough to pay for the enlargement and refoundation of his old college, changing its name from 'Gonville Hall' to 'Gonville and Caius College', as it is known today. To help pay for the upkeep of the new college, Caius endowed it with several large estates and added an entire new court at the cost of £1,834. He became master of the college in January 1559 and remained in the post until just before he died.[22]

Caius had first come to serve royalty as a physician when he was summoned to Henry VIII's court from his practice in Shrewsbury in Shropshire. There he had been studying cases of the mysterious 'sweating sickness' and writing a paper on the subject that was published as *An Account of the Sweating Sickness in England* in 1556, by which time the disease was fading from history, if only he'd known it. Having been a court physician during the reign of Henry VIII, he remained to serve both Edward VI and Mary Tudor, but Elizabeth I dismissed him because he was a devout Roman Catholic at her now Protestant court.

In 1557 he erected a monument in St Paul's Cathedral, London, to the memory of his fellow court physician and predecessor as president of the College of Physicians, Thomas Linacre. In 1564, he was given a grant by Gonville and Caius College to take the bodies of two malefactors annually for dissection, making him a pioneer in advancing the new science of anatomy in England. He designed and presented a silver caduceus, the medical symbol of Asculapius' staff entwined with snakes, sometimes seen today as the sign for a pharmacy. It still belongs to Caius College as part of its insignia, although he first gave it to the College of Physicians and afterwards presented the college with a replacement.

Caius died at his London home by St Bartholomew's Hospital on the 29 July 1573, but his body was brought to Cambridge for burial in the chapel of Gonville and Caius, under the monument that he had designed for himself.

The Health of the Tudor Monarchs

Both Thomas Linacre and John Caius were royal physicians at the Tudor court, but what kind of health problems afflicted the monarchs? Although the chroniclers of the time wrote in some detail about Henry VIII's physical condition, little could be said of any negative aspects of the king's health. Health bulletins had to be positive and encouraging, as if his majesty would live forever, otherwise a physician could have been in trouble. To mention any signs of deterioration in the king's condition was regarded as an act of treason.

In 1513, Henry VIII (r. 1509–47) suffered from an unidentified skin disease and, soon after, was afflicted by a mild attack of smallpox. He was also plagued by recurrent headaches.[23] Otherwise, he must have seemed the epitome of youthful good health. At six feet two inches tall, the king stood head and shoulders above most of his court. He had an athletic physique and excelled at sports, regularly showing off his prowess in the jousting arena.

Having inherited the good looks of his grandfather Edward IV, in 1515 Henry was described as 'the handsomest potentate I have ever set eyes on' and later as an 'Adonis with an extremely fine calf to his leg, his complexion very fair ... and a round face so very beautiful, that it would become a pretty woman'.[24] Records show that the king suffered a bout of quartan fever (malaria) in 1521, at a time when the disease was prevalent, especially in marshy areas of south-east England[25] – places ideal not only for the infected mosquitoes to breed but also for falconry and hawking, pastimes enjoyed by the king. Henry seems to have made a full recovery and continued to take part in tournaments, archery competitions, bowling and real (royal) tennis.

All this changed in 1536 when the king – then in his mid-forties – suffered a serious wound to his leg while jousting. This never healed completely and became ulcerous, which left Henry increasingly incapacitated. Four years later, it would seem that he had taken to drowning his sorrows in drink and comforting himself with prodigious amounts of rich food, with the result that his waistline expanded from a fairly trim thirty-two inches to an enormous fifty-two inches. In the months preceding his death, he was forced to resort to being winched onto his horse. Despite the artists who painted his many portraits being scrupulous in not showing any sign of his swollen leg and bandaging, sadly for Henry, it is these images of the corpulent old king that have become most famous.

Some sources suggest the king may have had syphilis,[26] and while this would explain his violent mood swings, ulcerated legs and even an abnormality beside his nose, others point out that an endocrine (hormonal) problem would also explain his symptoms. There is no evidence that Henry was given the new mercury treatment for syphilis – invented by Paracelsus – but whether this indicates the absence of the disease or the fact that English doctors had not yet learned of the treatment is impossible to say.

Brewer suggests that the king may have had a pituitary abnormality (basophil adenoma) and hyper-function of the suprarenal glands that lie just above the kidneys, known today as Cushing's disease.[27] In these cases, the patient becomes obese, his face bloated. He becomes 'markedly aggressive and quarrelsome with recurrent headaches' and suffers a loss of sexual function (virilism).[28] This seems to fit what we know of Henry's health problems in his later years. Other experts think that type 2 diabetes could have added to his woes. Henry died at Westminster on the night of 27/28 January 1547 of renal (kidney) and hepatic (liver) failure, aggravated by his obesity.[29] He was fifty-five.

Edward VI (r. 1547–53) was only ten-years-old when he succeeded his father and all his life he had been cosseted and protected from infections. Anyone in the prince's household who became unwell was sent away; any member of his staff who had cause to visit the filthy city of London, where diseases were rife, was obliged to spend time in quarantine before rejoining the prince's company. The royal apartments were regularly given a thoroughly good spring clean. Despite, or perhaps because of, this regime to protect Edward from any contagion, he suffered a bout of smallpox, or more possibly measles, in April 1552 and from that time his health declined. Edward himself wrote, 'I fell sike of the measles and the smallpookes.'[30] He was still very weak in Christmas 1552, and Brewer points out that 'measles is apt to be followed by pulmonary complications, even in a fit person'. We know that his grandfather Henry VII may have died of pulmonary tuberculosis and the boy's uncle Prince Arthur had definitely died of the disease in his mid-teens, so it appears that the Tudor menfolk were rather susceptible to it. During the following spring, it became obvious to the royal physicians that the young king was dying of consumption (tuberculosis). On his physicians' orders, he was moved to Greenwich (now in South-East London, but then in the rural countryside) where the air was healthy and free of filthy miasmas. By now, Edward was emaciated and coughing up blood-tinged sputum. Treasonous or not, an honest medical bulletin was released on the subject of the king's health:

> The physicians are all now agreed that he is suffering from a suppurative tumour on the lung. He is beginning to break out in ulcers [possibly bedsores]; he is vexed with a harsh and continuous cough, his body is dry and burning, his belly is swollen [possibly tuberculous peritonitis], he has a slow fever upon him that never leaves him.[31]

On 6 July 1553, Edward whispered his last prayer and died. He was only fifteen years old.

Edward was succeeded by his half-sister, Mary Tudor (r. 1553–58). At the time of her accession and her subsequent marriage to Philip II, King of Spain, at Winchester on 25 July 1554, Mary's health seemed good. Soon after the wedding, although she was already thirty-eight years old, Mary believed she was pregnant. It proved to be a phantom pregnancy and was followed by unspecified gastric and intestinal troubles. This spate of ill health was followed by what seems to have been another phantom pregnancy, but was in fact the early symptoms of the ovarian cancer that eventually killed the queen in November 1558. However, one source, *The Life of Mary*, which may be contemporary, but wasn't published until 1682, stated that the queen 'fell into a fever which, increasing little by little, at last put an end to her life, which fever at that time raged in most of England and swept away a great number of people'.[32] This is a reference to the 'sweating sickness', which may have been the ultimate cause of Mary's death.

The next and last Tudor monarch, Elizabeth I, certainly had a longer life than her half-siblings, but she too had her health problems. Despite these, she was generally very active, an accomplished horsewoman who rode daily up until the last months of her life. She would stand for hours in council meetings without tiring, much to the anguish of some of her elderly councillors who could not sit while their monarch stood. However, in 1559 Elizabeth suffered a recurrent fever which may have been a bout of malaria.[33] We heard in chapter 6 that the queen contracted smallpox in 1562, but throughout her life she seemed to suffer from debilitating headaches – sometimes at remarkably convenient moments, such as when Queen Mary demanded her presence at court.

Throughout her life, Elizabeth was plagued by toothache and tooth decay, but her physicians were too wary to suggest she have the offending molars extracted. One of her courtiers volunteered to have his bad teeth removed in the queen's presence, so she could see that the process wasn't so awful after all. The queen relented and permitted the offending royal teeth to be extracted.

During Elizabeth's reign, the royal medical staff was small, perhaps because the queen regarded any mention of illness as a weakness in itself, but the members of this select group were brought from all branches of medicine. Among her physicians were Lancelot Browne; Roger Gifford, a president of the College of Physicians; Robert Jacob; Edward Lister, the 'physician-in-ordinary'; Richard Master, also a president of the College of Physicians; and Roger Marbeck, who was as much a sea-roving adventurer as a physician. There was also Roderigo López, a Portuguese Jew who was appointed as Elizabeth's chief physician in 1586. Unfortunately for the queen's peace of mind, in 1594, López was arrested, accused of being involved in a plot to murder her. Even under interrogation and torture he protested his innocence, but he was tried, found guilty and hanged at Tyburn outside the City of London.[34] Elizabeth was never convinced of her physician's guilt, but Shakespeare is thought to have based his character 'Shylock' in *The Merchant of Venice* on Dr López.

The queen's surgeons seem to have been less suspect and

included John Woodall and William Clowes, both of whom had been surgeons to the army. Some sources give credit to Woodall as having been the first to use citrus juice as a cure for scurvy. And finally, the queen employed as her toothache specialist, general heath consultant, astrologer and heretical mystic John Dee. Dee gave his personal regimen for good health as 'eight hours a day study; two hours eating and four hours sleeping'.[35]

In March 1603, now sixty-nine years old, Elizabeth became quite unwell, in low spirits and depressed. She retired to her favourite home, Richmond Palace, upriver from London in the pleasant Surrey countryside. Stubborn as always, she wouldn't allow her doctors to examine her, insisting that she wasn't ill. She refused to go to her bed to rest and instead stood for hours on end, just occasionally relenting to rest in a chair. As her condition became worse and she still wouldn't go to bed, her ladies spread cushions on the floor for her. Eventually, the queen gave in and lay down on them. She spent almost four days lying on the floor, barely speaking a word except to insist she would not go to bed. Even Elizabeth could not deny death indefinitely, but only when she had grown so weak and speechless that she was unable to argue with her servants did they succeed in putting her to bed. Soft music was played to soothe her and her councillors gathered around.[36]

The cause of her death cannot be confirmed because there was never a post-mortem. She may have died of septicaemia (blood poisoning), possibly caused by years of application of the white make-up known as ceruse – a poisonous mixture of white lead and vinegar. If the final cause was septicaemia, Elizabeth's bad teeth may have contributed. The queen may have had a tooth abscess and, in the days before efficient antibiotics, there was the possibility that it might become life threatening. An example of a severe tooth abscess complication is Ludwig's angina, a serious form of cellulitis which inflames the tissues of the floor of the mouth. In extreme cases, this condition can close the air pathway and cause suffocation. It certainly makes speech very difficult, as well as eating and drinking – symptoms that affected the queen. Infection can then spread to the chest area, with serious implications for the heart and lungs. If the abscess doesn't drain, it may lead to sepsis, a whole-body infection that can cause limb loss, organ dysfunction and death.[37] Her physicians, surgeons and even her 'Merlin', John Dee, could do nothing to stave off the inevitable. Elizabeth I died on 24 March 1603, the last of the Tudor dynasty.

Ambroise Paré (1510–90)

On the Continent, the years spanned by Elizabeth's reign had witnessed endless wars, leading to some new innovations, particularly in battlefield surgery. The Frenchman Ambroise Paré, like many surgeons, gained much of his surgical experience as a result of war. Having served his apprenticeship to a barber-surgeon, one day in 1536, at the very beginning of his military career, there was a shortage of oil for cauterising the wounds of amputees and other injured men. It was common practice at the time for surgeons to seal wounds with boiling oil – an excruciating procedure which often failed to keep out infection, which it was supposed to do. As the newest recruit, Paré was reluctant to complain about having no oil, so he took the very risky step – both in terms of his future career with the army and the lives of the soldiers in his care – of inventing his own method of sealing the wounds. Instead of using oil, he made a tincture of egg yolk, turpentine and oil of roses and applied that to the men's injuries, but he wrote later that

> I could not sleep all that night, for I was troubled in mind and the dressing ... which I judged unfit, troubled my thoughts and I feared that next day I should find them dead, or at the point of death by the poison [infection] of the wound, whom I had not dressed with the scalding oil.[38]

The following morning, to his amazement, the soldiers who had been treated with the tincture were in a much better condition than those who had been treated with boiling oil.[39] Paré kept his job and continued to serve with the French army for thirty years, thanks, probably, to the antiseptic properties of the turpentine in his mixture. As his career progressed, Paré refused to use cauterisation to seal the limb stumps after amputation. In this case, he reverted to the use of ligatures to tie off the blood vessels, just as Galen had done for the Roman gladiators. Cauterising with red-hot irons didn't always stop the loss of blood and the shock of its application was sometimes enough to kill the patient. Although Paré's procedure was less painful for the patient than cauterisation, the ligatures themselves could introduce infection, complications and death, so were not always an unqualified success nor frequently adopted by other surgeons. For his new technique, he designed the *bec de corbin* or 'crow's beak', a predecessor of modern haemostats (arterial forceps to clamp the blood vessels). Paré detailed the technique in his 1564 book *Treatise on Surgery*. During his work with amputees, Paré noted the pain they experienced as sensations in the 'phantom' amputated limb. He believed that these phantom pains occur in the brain and not in the remnants of the limb – as medical opinion agrees today.[40] Paré designed prosthetic limbs for his amputee patients and also invented some ocular prostheses: artificial eyes which he made from enamelled gold, silver, porcelain and glass.

However, although some of Paré's ideas may have been new to the medical profession, other useful knowledge had its origins in old wives' tales. Paré put at least one of these to good effect:

One of the Marshall of Montejan's kitchen boys fell by chance into a cauldron of oil being almost boiling hot. I being called to dress him, went to the next apothecary's to fetch refrigerating medicines commonly used in this case. There was present by chance a certain old country woman who, hearing that I desired medicines for a burn, persuaded me at the first dressing, that I should lay [there]to raw onions beaten with a little salt, for so I should hinder the breaking out of blisters or pustules, as she had found by certain and frequent experience.[41]

Instead of dismissing the countrywoman's advice out of hand, as other medical professionals may well have done, Paré decided the remedy might be worth trying. The next day, he reported that where he had put the onions the boy's body was free of blisters, but other areas, untreated with onions, were badly blistered. Shortly after this experiment, it happened that a member of Montejan's guard was severely injured when his gunpowder flask caught fire. The man's face and hands were 'grievously burnt'. Again, Paré treated the patient with the onion mixture but, because he regarded it as an experimental procedure, he only applied it to parts of the man's face; the rest he treated with 'the medicines usually applied to burns'. When he changed the dressing, he discovered, as in the first case, the onions had prevented blistering and excoriation (skin peeling), although the other areas, treated in the normal way, were 'troubled with both', whereby he wrote, 'I gave credit to the [onion] Medicine'.[42] He published his first book, *The Method of Curing Wounds Caused by Arquebus and Firearms*, in 1545, refuting the idea of his contemporaries that gunpowder was poisonous and this poison caused the wounded to die, no matter what was done by the surgeon. Theriac – that supposed antidote to all poisons – was still being used to treat gunshot wounds.

Paré was also interested in the new anatomical ideas being introduced by Andreas Versalius and others in the field. Paré developed a number of instruments and artificial limbs, and introduced new ideas in obstetrics, reintroducing the practice of 'podalic version', a procedure in which the position of a foetus in the uterus (usually a second twin that is presenting transversely or obliquely) is altered so that its feet will emerge first at birth, giving it a chance of survival. He also introduced the lancing of infants' gums during teething, believing this would aid the emerging teeth. At the time, it was thought babies could die because the teeth 'lacked a pathway' through the gums. The controversial practice was continued until near the end of the nineteenth century when, thankfully, it went out of fashion.

In 1552, Paré left the army and went into royal service, attending the French king, Henry II (r. 1519–59). Able as he was, Paré couldn't cure the king when he sustained a fatal blow to his head during a tournament in 1590, but he continued serving the kings of France: Henry II, Francis II, Charles IX and Henry III. According to one of the king's ministers, Sully, Paré was a Huguenot (a Protestant in Roman Catholic France) and on 24 August 1572, the day of the infamous St Bartholomew's Day Massacre, Paré's life was saved when King Charles IX locked him in a clothes closet. It's a great story, but there is no evidence that the royal surgeon was anything other than a devout Roman Catholic. Paré died in Paris in 1590 from natural causes, at the age of seventy-nine.

With groundbreaking innovators like Ambroise Paré now advancing the field of medicine during the sixteenth century, hopefully, progress would continue at an ever-increasing rate in the seventeenth. Was this the case, or did old ideas continue to hamper the advance of medical theory and practice? This will be the subject of the next chapter.

12

PROGRESS IN MEDICINE?

Further treatment was made difficult by the death of the King.

Sir Charles Scarburgh's diary, 1685

Although it is not easy to realise the fact, the practitioners of the medieval period had contributed a great deal to the field of medical knowledge. There was progress in surgery, medical chemistry, dissection and practical medicine. While there might not be any monumental steps forward, they certainly laid the ground work for later discoveries. There was a slow but constant progression in the way that medicine was studied and practised. Surgeons in particular added practical knowledge to the theoretical approach of the universities, and oral traditions and ancient texts were being supplemented by contemporary writings on new ideas and findings.

There had been an early attempt at vivisection made in 1474 in an effort to observe what went on inside the body of a living man. The evidence comes from *The History of Louis XI*, written by John of Troyes. According to this writer, a French archer was to be hanged in Paris for robbing churches. The archer suffered from colic, the stone and pains in his side, as did one of King Louis's favourite courtiers. A group of Parisian physicians and surgeons suggested to the king that it would be useful to see the inner workings of a living body in order to find the root cause of these problems and the condemned archer, about to die anyway, would be the ideal specimen. Louis gave his permission and the archer was offered a royal pardon if he agreed to let the doctors make their drastic internal examination:

> Which opening and incision was accordingly done on the body of the said archer and the place of the said maladies having been sought out and examined, his bowels were replaced and he was sewn up again. And by the king's command the wound was well dressed so that he was perfectly healed within a fortnight.[1]

With his pardon and some money, the archer was free to go. What the account doesn't tell us is what the doctors learned from this intrusive surgery, which must have been excruciating for the specimen. Neither do we hear whether either the archer or the courtier benefitted from any discoveries made.

Advances in [Al]chemical Studies

Plants were still the main source of medieval remedies, but at the beginning of the sixteenth century medical chemistry became more prominent, with the adaptation of alchemical processes to the preparation of medicines. As methods grew more refined and technical – for example, the process of distillation – remedies could be made more potent and pure because there was a way to remove any nonessential ingredients and purify the important ones. The use of alcohol as a solvent for some of the vital ingredients that wouldn't dissolve in water was another advance. For example, Paracelsus had discovered that the active ingredients of opium dissolve far more readily in alcohol (to make laudanum) than in water; vanilla extract can also be dissolved in alcohol, but not in water.

Some of the steps along the way towards the new science of chemistry certainly had elements of hocus-pocus and black magic about them, with their continuing quest for the Philosopher's Stone and the Elixir of Life. George Ripley was born at Ripley, near Harrogate in Yorkshire, in the early fifteenth century. He studied alchemy in Rome, Louvain and on the island of Rhodes. While on Rhodes, he created gold for the Knights of St John, giving them £100,000 a year – so he claimed, but of course the process was far too involved and secret to be divulged.

In 1471, George was a canon at Bridlington Priory where it was noted how the fumes and stink from his still-room (laboratory) annoyed the prior and brethren of the community. He wrote books on the alchemical arts: *On the Philosophers' Stone and the Phoenix* was a rewriting of earlier authors from the thirteenth and fourteenth centuries, so wasn't too controversial. However, his *Compound of Alchemy or the Twelve Gates Leading to the Discovery of the Philosophers' Stone*, the first alchemical text written in English, in 1471, was dedicated to King Edward IV, just to be on the safe side, and his Latin *Medulla alchemiae* or *Marrow of Alchemy* of 1476 was dedicated to the Archbishop of York. The twelve gates were the various chemical techniques then known (for example, calcination, condensation and sublimation) and it was these processes that paved the way for modern chemists.

To give you some idea of the lengths to which an alchemist would go to disguise his secret formulae, this is Ripley's colourful description from his *Compound of Alchemy* of the making of the Elixir of Eternal Life – the alchemists' other goal in addition to the Philosophers' Stone – complete with a zoo full of metaphorical creatures:

Pale & black with false citrine, imperfect white & red,
The peacock's feathers in colour gay, the rainbow which
    shall overgo,

The spotted panther, the lion green, the crow's bill blue as
    lead,
These shall appear before the perfect white and many other
    mo'e.
And after the perfect white, grey, false citrine also,
And after these then shall appear the body red invariable,
Then hast thou a medicine of the third order of his own
    kind multiplicable.[2]

Apparently, the green lion symbolises the element mercury, the
lion often being referred to as 'devouring the sun', i.e. gold.
Mercury will dissolve gold (and silver) to form an amalgam which
can be used for gilding other metals. The alchemists believed
mercury was *the* element, a component of all other known metals
which made it possible to turn them liquid when heated. Because
it was so important, it was symbolised by the most illustrious
animal, the lion, but why green? I haven't been able to discover the
answer to this so far. Mercury was also known to alchemists as the
doorkeeper, May dew, mother egg and the bird of Hermes – just a
few of its exotic names.

When George Ripley died around 1490, he was rich – far richer
than a humble canon ought to be – so folk believed he must have
succeeded in making gold but, on his deathbed, he confessed
to having wasted his whole lifetime in fruitless pursuits, urging
that his writings should all be burned, seeing they were merely
speculation, not based on valid experiments at all. Of course, his
books weren't destroyed. After all, George had got rich by some
means, and if not by alchemy then how?

Thomas Norton was a Bristol man from a respected family.
His grandfather had been mayor of Bristol. Born around 1433,
Thomas did a kind of correspondence course in alchemy with
George Ripley and, aged twenty-eight, spent forty days studying
at Ripley's side. Thomas was supposed to have succeeded in

making the Elixir of Life – twice – only to have it stolen from him, once by a servant and once by the wife of neighbouring Bristol merchant. According to his great-grandson Samuel Norton (also an alchemist), Thomas was a member of King Edward IV's privy chamber. This is quite possible. Edward certainly took a serious interest in alchemy, probably because the manufacture of gold would have done his perennially depleted coffers a world of good (he may even have 'dabbled' himself). In 1477, Thomas published a book called the *Ordinal of Alchemy* which was still in print in 1652, but he didn't dare declare his authorship openly, concealing his name by encoding it in a cipher.

In 1479, Thomas accused the then mayor of Bristol of treason. In the course of enquiries, Thomas's own life came under examination and was found to be anything but blameless: he frequented taverns, skipped church and played tennis on Sundays. The charges against the mayor were dropped; the accusations of a backslider like Thomas would not have carried weight in court.

However weird and baffling the works of men like George Ripley and Thomas Norton may seem to us today, they opened many doors for medieval physicians because new compounds were being made, often accidentally, in their determination to discover the Philosopher's Stone. Increasingly, they were finding substances derived from mineral sources, some of which found their way onto an ever-growing list of possible medical remedies.

William Harvey (1578–1657)

We have already heard a little about William Harvey, but a closer look at his career shows the struggle physicians were having, trying to break away from the classical traditions of medieval medicine. He was born at Folkestone in Kent, son of the four-time mayor of the town. At the age of ten, young William was sent to boarding school in Canterbury, to the King's School attached to the cathedral, where he got a good grounding in Greek and Latin, the language he would use later to write the books that would make his name. In 1593, he went to Gonville and Caius College, Cambridge, graduating in 1597. He was determined to continue his medical studies and went on to the University of Padua – reputedly the best school of medicine in Europe. Galileo was a teacher there and, without a doubt, it was here that Harvey's interest in the 'scientific method' crystallised. The scientific method was all about first-hand knowledge, finding out by doing the experiments and not by reading the old textbooks. Like the other students, Harvey was aware of Galileo's new approach to teaching and he learned from dissection and anatomical observation. For two and a half years he studied under the guidance of a celebrated anatomist and teacher, known as Fabricius, in the now famous Anatomy Theatre, still to be seen at the university in Padua.

Harvey saw that there were problems posed by the function of the beating heart and the properties of the blood passing through it. His tutor, Fabricius, went into great detail on the workings of the other organs and even dissected out the valves in the veins to demonstrate how they allowed blood to flow in only one direction. Yet he skirted around the action and purpose of the heart and Harvey determined to correct the omission. As a student, Harvey was popular and was elected Conciliarius, or leader of the English students in Padua, but, like doctors throughout history, apparently his handwriting was terrible.

Now fully qualified, Harvey returned to London in 1603. In order to practise he had to have a licence, and on 4 May 1603, aged twenty-five, he presented himself to the Censors of the College of Physicians for examination and was given his licence. After that, his career took off. He was admitted as a member of the College of Physicians in April 1604 and married Elizabeth Browne, the daughter of Lancelot Browne. Browne was an important man, a royal physician to Queen Elizabeth I (who had been buried at Westminster the week before Harvey applied for his licence) and then to King James I and his queen, Anne of Denmark. He was also a senior Fellow of the College of Physicians and having these connections in high places did young Harvey no harm at all. Two years after being elected a Fellow of the College in 1607, he was appointed Physician to St Bartholomew's Hospital, becoming Lumleian Lecturer at the College of Physicians in 1616.

At the time, St Bartholomew's had about 200 beds in twelve wards and Harvey's duties consisted of attending on at least one day a week in the main hall. Here, sitting at the table in front of the great fireplace – the fire was supplied with wood from the forest at Windsor, a privilege granted by Henry III over 300 years before – Harvey would see and interview the walking patients. He received an annual salary of £25 with £2 extra for his livery (a food and clothing allowance) and a further £8 in lieu of not living in the official physician's residence on site, since he preferred to live with his wife in nearby St Martin's.

In 1612, 'a whole college of physicians' was summoned to attend King James's most important minister, Robert Cecil. Cecil was 'laid low by reason of the weakness of his body', a reference to a deformity described unflatteringly by one enemy as a 'wry neck, a crooked back and a splay foot', another referring to him as 'a hunchbacked dwarf'. The king's physician, Sir Thomas Mayerne, was confident of success in treating Cecil but couldn't decide on a correct diagnosis. In the end, it was Harvey and his surgeon, Joseph Fenton, summoned from St Bartholomew's, who did 'most good' in treating the invalid although they couldn't cure him. He died two months later of what was probably scurvy. Harvey held his office at St Bartholomew's for thirty-four years, being displaced for political reasons by Oliver Cromwell's regime when it held sway in London. The regime disliked and mistrusted the physician's royal connections.

Lecturing at the College of Physicians, he was expected to use real corpses to demonstrate the organs and functions of the body. This could be a problem because only the bodies of hanged criminals were allowed to be dissected and the supply was intermittent and unreliable, not to mention too scarce for the lecturers who needed them. Also, before the days of refrigeration, particularly in warm weather, the corpses quickly deteriorated and began to stink. Harvey had a series of three lectures that could be delivered at short notice, one after the other, each lasting about an hour. The first looked at the external bodily form and function, the second examined the chest cavity, heart, lungs, etc. and the third lecture was on the head, brain and nervous system, all done in three hours.

He was always cutting up bodies of animals to increase his knowledge and hone his skills in dissection, having the king's permission to use deer killed in the royal park at Windsor. He was pleased whenever an injured animal was brought to him because only a live animal could provide the evidence that he needed to prove his developing theories on blood circulation. During his career, he performed dissections on cats, chickens, guinea pigs, seals, snakes, moles, rats, frogs, fish, pigeons, an ostrich, his wife's parrot, a pet monkey, a human foetus, his father and his sister.

The Heart of the Matter

Harvey worked out how arterial blood flowed from the left ventricle of the heart to the aorta and was then distributed through this major blood vessel and on, via the arteries, to all parts of the body. Having now changed from arterial to venous blood, it was then carried through the veins, via the vena cava, back to the right atrium of the heart from which it flowed down into the right ventricle. The right ventricle pumped the blood into the pulmonary artery for the short trip to the lungs, where the dark venous blood was refreshed with oxygen and the carbon dioxide removed, turning it into bright-scarlet arterial blood that returned, through the pulmonary vein, to the left atrium or auricle and down into the left ventricle to begin the cycle again.

The part of the cycle that remained a mystery for now was how the arterial blood, having reached the outer parts of the body and done its job, re-entered the veins to return to the heart. Microscopes had only just been invented and Harvey didn't use one. Even if he had, the fine capillaries that completed the circulation may not have been visible under the very early microscopes, but Harvey was clever enough to deduce that these tiny blood vessels must exist.

A number of doctors before Harvey had already decided that Galen's ancient teaching was wrong, that the liver did not send the blood out around the body. The theory was that the blood arrived in the right side of the heart and seeped through invisible pores in the cardiac septum that divided it from the left ventricle of the heart. In the left ventricle air was mixed with the blood, but no one had ever found a single pore in the septum – because there weren't any, of course. In 1553, Michael Servetius, a Spanish doctor and theologian, published *Christianismi Restitutio*, a work that rejected this idea and earned him death at the stake for heresy. His book is reckoned today to be the rarest in the world because the Inquisition ordered every copy to be burned, but one at least must have survived because we know it contains, almost as an aside, the suggestion of pulmonary circulation and a denial that the septum was porous.

Harvey's great achievement was to complete the solution to the problem, with the supporting evidence from his experiments to confirm his hypothesis. He suggested that the heart was a pump, worked by muscular force; he observed the phenomenon of 'systole' – the contraction of the walls of the heart at the moment they force out the blood – and 'diastole' – the relaxing of the walls to allow blood to refill the heart. Together with his knowledge of the valves in the heart and veins, as well as the observation that veins swelled below a ligature, he was able to work out the direction of blood flow and the mechanics of the cardiovascular system. The heart prompted Harvey into raptures. Other organs he described with clinical detachment, but this is what he said of the heart: 'The empire of the heart is the principal part of all ... the citadel and home of heat, household god of the edifice [body]; the fountain, conduit, head of life: All things are united in the heart!'[3]

Harvey had been telling his students about circulation for some twelve years, but it was only when he published his findings that the medical profession took notice. The book was published in Frankfurt in 1628. Written in Latin and entitled *Exercitatio anatomica de motu cordis et sanguinis in animalibus* (*On the Motion of the Heart and Blood in Animals*), it had two full-page diagrams to explain the text and remains one of the greatest discoveries in physiology. Not surprisingly, there were some in the medical profession, especially on the Continent, who disputed his discovery and dismissed him as 'crackbrained'. For a time he actually feared physical injury to himself, so vehement was the envy of a few others, but he continued, patiently and good-naturedly, to argue his case. All the time his reputation was increasing, as well as his wealth, as more and more people wanted to be treated by the eminent physician, although his contemporary John Aubrey tells us he lost a few of his more conservative clients, who disapproved of his newfangled crazy ideas.

In 1618, Harvey had been appointed physician-extraordinary to James I and, when the king died in 1625, he was called to defend the reputation of the monarch's favourite, the Duke of Buckingham, who was accused of having poisoned the king. The physician's testimony exonerated the duke. It seems that James had been suffering from a chronic chest infection for some while; modern diagnosis suggests this was fibroid tuberculosis of the lungs. In the spring of 1625, London was once again in the grip of the plague, so the royal court removed to Theobalds, a fine manor house near Hatfield in Hertfordshire, for the benefit of the king's health. But the hoped for improvement didn't happen. James became seriously ill, suffering recurrent attacks of fever (described as the 'ague') and occasional convulsions. He grew steadily worse, saying, 'I shall never see London again', and got no relief from the various applications and drinks prescribed by his physicians.

The Duke of Buckingham suggested a remedy that he said he had tried himself and found to be 'of great medicinal value'. James refused to take the white powder at first but, at Buckingham's insistence, he eventually agreed to take it in a little wine, only to be suddenly afflicted with 'violent fluxes of the belly'. At the same time, he allowed Buckingham's mother to apply a salve on a plaster to his breast, whereupon he grew faint, short of breath and in great agony. The smell of the salve attracted the attention of the physicians who rushed into the chamber, snatched away the offending plaster and exclaimed the king was being poisoned. 'Poisoning me!' James is said to have cried out before fainting away in horror. Buckingham then threatened the physicians with banishment from the court 'if they kept not good tongues in their heads'. One of the physicians, George Eglington, observed that 'in the mean time, the King's body and head swelled above measure, his hair with the skin of his head stuck to the pillow, his nails became loose upon his fingers and toes, the extremities of which became blackened.' These could be symptoms of poisoning by either white arsenic or sublimate of mercury but, since both substances were reckoned as legitimate medications at that time, it seems more likely that James was the victim of an accidental overdose rather than an intentional act of poisoning. Whatever the case, the king went rapidly downhill after that, developing severe diarrhoea and becoming seriously dehydrated, which caused his death on the 25 March 1625. As we have heard, Harvey was instrumental in exonerating Buckingham of complicity in the king's death, so either he believed the remedies to have been innocuous after all, or else thought it was the case that James had been overdosed by mistake. Whatever the truth, within a few weeks, Harvey received a 'gift' of the princely sum of £100 from the new king, Charles I, 'for his pains and attendance about the person of his Majesty's late dear father, of happy memory, in time of his sickness'.

The new king's generosity confirmed Harvey's special position at Charles's side where he would remain the most loyal and devoted servant to the king during one of the roughest reigns in English history. Charles I and Harvey became good friends and whenever the king travelled, Harvey would go with him. On a state visit to Scotland, he used the opportunity to visit the Bass Rock to study the colony of breeding gannets, continuing his interests as a naturalist from his student days, being intrigued by the discovery that the guillemots seemed to have cemented their eggs to the cliff to keep them from falling off the precipitous ledges, into the sea. He wrote up accounts of his observations and, whenever the chance offered, he would dissect a bird or animal to see how the internal organs were arranged, looking at over sixty different species during his lifetime.

In 1634, four Lancashire women were accused of witchcraft and Harvey was appointed to lead the examining committee consisting of ten midwives and seven surgeons. They found there was nothing unnatural in their bodies and the women were pardoned, having undergone a humiliating, personal inspection before and at the hands of the committee. However, he wasn't above reproach: a man described as an 'impudent barber-surgeon' claimed Harvey was responsible for malpractice on a maidservant who subsequently died. He defended himself rigorously and his reputation remained intact. Another celebrated case for him was the post-mortem carried out on a Shropshire labourer, Thomas Parr, who was supposed to have lived for 152 years and nine months. Of particular interest was the fact that, already aged well over 100 years, Parr had been prosecuted for fornication and the king wished to know whether the man had actually still been capable of such a sin. Harvey was able to report that the post-mortem revealed the ancient genitalia to have been 'entirely consistent with a prosecution for fornication'.

Ever the experimentalist, Harvey liked to get the king involved in his 'discoveries'. One such discovery, made in 1640, was the Viscount Hugh Montgomery, a young Irish nobleman 'with a good complexion and habit of body'. Harvey brought the viscount before Charles I and opened his shirt to reveal a metal plate attached to the lower left side of the lad's chest. He removed the plate to show the king a hole in his chest into which Charles was invited to insert his fingers. He felt a 'fleshy part sticking out which was driven in and out by a reciprocal motion'. Others had assumed this was the breathing lung beneath a membrane of scar tissue, but the ever-observant Harvey realised the movement coincided not with the young man's breathing but with his pulse. Therefore, what the king could feel was the heart beating. Harvey was delighted to demonstrate this to Charles, justifying the theory he had published earlier in the king's name. Montgomery explained how the hole had been caused when he'd broken his ribs as a child. The injury had become infected for a long time and had eventually healed, leaving the hole that never closed over. Every morning his valet would cleanse the hole and cover it with the specially made metal plate to protect it. Otherwise the young viscount was as fit and healthy as any other eighteen-year-old lad.

As the king's personal physician, Harvey was involved in the English Civil War, although he had little interest in either the drama or the politics. While the king was raising his standard and his army was assembling at Nottingham in August 1642, Harvey went off to visit a doctor friend in Derby, Percival Willoughby, recording that they talked about uterine diseases. This subject would be relevant to his next book. He followed the king to Oxford and was appointed Warden of Merton College. While at the university, he took the opportunity to carry out research, concentrating on experiments in embryology by studying the development of chicks in hens' eggs. He was fascinated by fertility, perhaps because he and his wife Elizabeth had no children. Meanwhile, London was a stronghold of the Parliamentarians and he was bitterly upset when news came that a riotous mob had attacked his apartment in the king's palace at Whitehall and ransacked it, burning all his books and papers relevant to his medical practice, work and experiments.

Further sad news reached him at Oxford in the winter of 1642, that his twin brothers, Matthew and Michael, were gravely ill in London. Matthew died just before Christmas and Harvey sent instructions for treating Michael. Unfortunately, by the time the physician's directive reached London in the middle of January, Michael was gone as well. In 1645 his wife, Elizabeth, died too, and the following year, after the surrender of Oxford in July 1646, Harvey fled north with King Charles, who gave himself up to the Scots. In January 1647, the Scots handed over the king to the forces of Oliver Cromwell and Harvey was told his services were no longer required. He was allowed to return to London where he lodged with one brother or another in their fine houses on the outskirts of the city. They had each become wealthy and successful merchants, particularly William's favourite brother Eliab, with whom he shared a great fondness for, if not an addiction to, the newly fashionable beverage of coffee. King Charles I was tried and executed in January 1649. Harvey was now broken and unhappy and virtually gave up practising medicine. However, he continued to conduct research into reproduction and embryology.

Studying Gynaecology

Harvey's second important book, *Exercitatio anatomica de generatione animalium* (*Anatomical Exercitations Concerning the Generation of Living Creatures*) was published in 1653. With the chapter on midwifery, he is said to have founded the modern study of gynaecology in this country because it was the first work on the subject written by an Englishman. According to Harvey, still writing in Latin, 'the younger, more giddy, and officious Midwives are to be rebuked' for intervening too actively in the birthing process 'lest they should seem unskilful at their trade'. In fact, he reckoned poor women, who couldn't afford to employ a properly trained midwife, were better off avoiding midwives altogether. This view was widely endorsed, particularly by Percival Willoughby, the physician Harvey had visited to discuss such matters while King Charles was at Nottingham in the summer of 1642. Willoughby wrote, 'I know but Dr Harvey's directions and method, the which I wish all midwives to observe and follow, and oft to read over and over again.'

Actually, Harvey's *De generatione* wouldn't have been much use to a midwife as it contained only a few comments relevant to human births, tacked onto the end of what was otherwise a scientific treatise. It wasn't meant to be a medical handbook and the first 362 pages dealt with every stage of development of a hen, in minute detail, from new laid egg to the hatched chicken. When he did get around to looking at human births, he quoted a number of novel cases he had come across during his years of practice, such as this example:

A certain Servant-Maid being gotten with Child by her Master who, to hide her knavery came to London in September, where she lay in by stealth: and being recovered again, returned home: but in December following, a new birth (for she had a Superfoetation) did proclaim the crime which she had cunningly concealed before.

A superfoetation was thought possible when a second conception occured during pregnancy while a foetus was already developing in the womb – so there were two babies, but not twins and, in this case, born three months apart. It is worth noting that in sixteenth-century society a maid being made pregnant by her master was seen as *her* evil-doing, not his.

On another occasion, Harvey was given some 'black little bones' produced by a mother following a successful birth. These he identified as the residue of a previous abortion. His book was well respected and critically acclaimed. After the publication of the English edition in 1653, it became widely read. One critic wrote, 'It was full of excellent learning and observation, despite the failure to explain how an embryo came to form without any sensible corporeal agent, by mere imagination, not of the brain, but of the womb.'

Harvey said that humans and other mammals reproduce by means of an egg fertilised by a sperm. With the invention of the microscope towards the end of the sixteenth century, Aristotle's and Galen's theories on the male and female 'contributions' to conception were discredited. It was now apparent that the woman produced 'eggs' and that they existed whether she took pleasure in sex or not – gone were the days of the 'necessary' orgasm. Men were now known to produce sperm in their semen and it was realised that this and the egg were the important elements in the process of fertilisation. These twin discoveries led to the theory of 'preformation' of the foetus in two forms. One camp, the ovists, believed that the egg contained a minute but fully formed baby, requiring the arrival of the male sperm only to trigger it into growth. The other group, the animalculists, disliking the idea of this trivial contribution on the part of the man, thought that a preformed individual – an 'animalcule' – existed in the head of the sperm and simply required the presence of the egg in the womb as something to provide it with nourishment and a place to grow. It would be another 200 years before microscopes were developed that could enable scientists to see the process of fertilisation taking place and observe the cellular changes in the ovum that gave rise to the foetus, disproving both theories.

Harvey's ability as a scientist and thinker was recognised by the Fellows in the College of Physicians when they elected him as their president in 1654, but they had left the accolade too late. He declined the honour on account of his old age and ill health, suffering from kidney stones and attacks of gout, treating the latter ailment by sitting with his feet in icy cold water. He described himself to a friend in a letter as 'not only ripe in years, but also a little weary and entitled to an honourable discharge'.

He had already paid for the building of a hall and library for the College of Physicians and given them his collection of medical books. Unfortunately, all his bequests – buildings and books – would be destroyed in the Great Fire of London in 1666. When Harvey awoke on 3 June 1657, he found he couldn't speak, a 'dead palsy' having taken his tongue. Instead of sending for a fellow physician, he sent for his apothecary, Sambroke of Blackfriars, who (in violation of College rules) let the blood in Harvey's tongue, but to no effect. He died soon after of a stroke at the age of seventy-nine, his passing helped, according to his old friend and fellow Royalist from Oxford, Dr Charles Scarburgh, by a powerful draught of opium.

There were a number of more personal bequests in his will. He left his father's farm on Romney Marsh to the College of Physicians and the family home in Folkestone to his Cambridge College, Gonville and Caius. He wanted his brother Eliab to have his best coffee pot, from which the two had shared so much of the expensive and exotic liquid, along with £20,000 – a colossal sum at the time – and he left his watch to his nephew. Incidentally, at the time, coffee was believed to have considerable medicinal properties of particular benefit to men, improving their libido among other things. Harvey also left £200 for the poor people of Folkestone, part of which sum went to found a Free School in the town that today is the Harvey Grammar School. William Harvey was buried in a vault, built by Eliab, at Hempstead Church in Essex, preceded by a procession from London attended by the Fellows of the

College of Physicians. His first biographer, the old gossip John Aubrey, who told us about Harvey's dreadful handwriting, helped to carry the lead-lined coffin. Ashford hospital, commissioned in 1977, is named after William Harvey and his statue stands at the entrance to the main building.

Among Harvey's successors was Thomas Sydenham. He was granted his licence to practise by the College of Physicians in 1663. His approach to medicine was revolutionary, but quite straightforward in that Sydenham insisted on accurate, clinical observations of a disease being noted down, the details of diagnosis to be accompanied by clear drawings and diagrams, if these were appropriate. Such record keeping was a real innovation and Sydenham soon had the opportunity to describe at first hand the virulence of the plague when the epidemic of 1665–66 struck London and south-eastern England. Unfortunately for him, one of his brave new ideas made Sydenham a laughing stock among many of his fellow physicians because he dared to disapprove of bloodletting as the universal cure-all, condoning its use in a few very particular cases only.

A Systematic Approach to Using Plants

Since medieval times, the trade in medicinal plants in London was still controlled by the Grocers' Company, as it had been for centuries. The apothecaries' business was concentrated in Bucklersbury in the city, an area famous for its herbal aroma. In 1617, the apothecaries broke away from the Grocers' Guild to form the Society of Apothecaries, claiming that

> very many empiricks and unskilled and ignorant men ... do abide in our city ... which are not well instructed in the art and mystery of Apothecaries but ... do make and compound many unwholesome, hurtful, deceitful, corrupt dangerous medicines.

In 1676, the apothecaries set up the Chelsea Physic Garden – now the second-oldest botanical garden in England after the one at Oxford – on land donated by Sir Hans Sloane. Here they grew as many plants as could fit into the fairly small site from among those which could survive the English climate or thrive in the glasshouses. The original purpose of the garden was to supply quality ingredients to the apothecaries of London, but it soon became a centre of experimentation and the search for new medicines – a process that goes on today.

Among the plants grown in the Physic Garden nowadays is the source of a relatively new treatment for childhood leukaemia: the Madagascan or rosy periwinkle, *Catharanthus roseus*.[4] It was discovered as a result of work done in the 1950s by the Canadian Dr Robert L. Noble and his colleagues.[5] This pretty plant from Madagascar looks rather like a pink Busy-Lizzie and gives us two very important cancer-fighting medicines: vinblastine and vincristine.

Traditional healers had used the rosy periwinkle for treating diabetes and this encouraged further study by western scientists. They couldn't find that it reduced sugar levels in the blood significantly, as they'd hoped, but it drastically lowered the white blood cell count. This led to the discovery of its anti-cancer properties. The drug vinblastine has helped increase the chance of surviving childhood leukaemia and lymphoma since its first trials in 1959 from 10 per cent to 95 per cent, while vincristine is used to treat Hodgkin's disease,[6] advanced testicular cancer and breast cancer.

As science improved and active ingredients were isolated and synthesised, the apothecary's art was increasingly replaced by the science of the pharmacist. Even today, seven out of ten of our medicines originate from herbal sources.[7]

Returning to the apothecaries of the sixteenth century, it is soon apparent that very little had changed since medieval times. William

Shakespeare, writing around 1600, included a description of an apothecary's shop in his play *Romeo and Juliet*. In act 5, scene 1, Romeo is considering where he can buy a potion to feign death:

> I do remember an apothecary –
> And hereabouts he dwells – which late I noted
> In tattered weeds, with overwhelming brows,
> Culling of simples. Meager were his looks,
> Sharp misery had worn him to the bones,
> And in his needy shop a tortoise hung,
> An alligator stuffed and other skins
> Of ill-shaped fishes; and about his shelves
> A beggarly account of empty boxes,
> Green earthen pots, bladders and musty seeds,
> Remnants of packthread and old cakes of roses,
> Were thinly scattered to make up a show.

We might have hoped this was an archaic image of such a shop, run by a professional, but that doesn't seem to have been the case. If we have any doubts, the case of a most illustrious patient, eighty-five years later, shows that musty seeds and the odd stuffed reptile were still available as treatments – and there was much worse besides.

King Charles II (r. 1660–85)

In 1685, King Charles II had the best medical attention money could buy and was treated by a team of the most distinguished physicians when he suffered what seems to have been a slight stroke. The king's ordeal began at eight o'clock on the morning of 2 February at his palace in Whitehall, London. Charles was about to have his daily shave when he suddenly cried out in pain and suffered a fit – most likely from a stroke that produced a brain seizure. One of his physicians, Edmund King, was summoned and applied what was considered 'emergency treatment', draining blood from a vein in the king's left arm. Meanwhile, messengers were sent to fetch the king's chief physician, Sir Charles Scarburgh.

'I flocked quickly to the King's assistance,' Scarburgh wrote later in his diary. After consulting with six of his colleagues, Scarburgh concluded that Charles was no better because Edmund King had taken insufficient blood, so Scarburgh drained an additional eight ounces (a little less than half a pint) by cupping, in which the king's shoulder was cut in three places and cupped to draw out the blood from his right arm. The king, who had lain senseless, now moved slightly and this was thought to be a good sign that he would benefit from the loss of more fluids from his body. Therefore, Scarburgh administered a 'volumous emetic' of poisonous antimony potassium tartrate (otherwise used as a caustic corrosive for dyeing cloth), rock salt, marshmallow leaves, violets, beetroot, camomile flowers, fennel seed, linseed, cardamom seed, cinnamon, saffron, cochineal and aloes. This caused violent retching and vomiting. Then the king was given an enema to 'extract more ill humours'. Having lost a significant amount of blood and vomited strenuously for an hour, he was then subjected to a bout of severe diarrhoea. Two hours later, with Charles unconscious and seeming to make little progress, his physicians decided that another enema should be administered as well as a laxative taken by mouth.

The king's head was then shaved and a blister raised on his scalp using plasters of cantharis, or Spanish fly. This substance is caustic and readily absorbed through the skin. It irritates the urinary tract, causing frequent urination and the further loss of fluids, but the physicians thought to draw the bad humours out from the brain, to be removed by lancing the blisters. A sneezing powder of poisonous white hellebore rhizome was given to further purge the brain and a powder of cowslip administered to strengthen it. The emetics were continued at frequent intervals and meanwhile a soothing drink was given, made of barley water, liquorice, sweet almonds, light wine, oil of wormwood, anise, thistle leaves, mint, rose and angelica. A plaster of pitch and pigeon dung was put on the king's feet, intended to draw any remaining ill humours away from his head.

The king regained consciousness, most likely because he was in agony, but Scarburgh saw this as proof that the treatments were working at last. This 'success' meant the procedures were continued with more bleeding and yet another, different, chemical emetic, followed by the administration of the most massive laxative yet, to 'keep the bowels open during the night'.

By now the unfortunate monarch should have been dead from dehydration, if not poisoning, yet on Tuesday morning, unbelievably, he was not only still breathing but alert. Scarburgh saw this as evidence of 'the blessing of God being approved by the application of proper and seasonable remedies' and eleven more physicians joined those already crowded into the royal bedchamber, each with their own 'infallible remedy' with which to treat the poor king. After examining Charles, they decided he would benefit from more bleeding, so they opened the veins in his neck and drained ten ounces of ill humours. Then they gave him to drink a julep with crushed melon seeds, manna, slippery elm, black cherry water, extract of lily-of-the-valley, peony, lavender, pearls dissolved in vinegar, gentian root, sugar, nutmeg and cloves. The slippery elm bark would have helped replace the mucous lining of his gut and could have given him some relief, but the lily-of-the-valley was yet another poison.

On Wednesday, the king suffered another seizure and so they bled him again and gave him forty drops of the extract of pulverised human skull, from an innocent man who had met a violent end. Charles slept fitfully, but at least he had no further seizures. On Thursday, exhausted and dehydrated by his physicians' continued treatments and in great pain, the king was bled again and given both oral laxatives and another enema. Then they administered the 'magic bullet' of the day: Jesuits' bark – quinine. Used to both prevent and treat malaria, it is nonetheless toxic in large doses. It wasn't appropriate in this case anyway and Scarburgh and his colleagues were perplexed when the king's condition became suddenly worse. Yet Thomas, Lord Fairfax, praised the king's physicians, saying, 'All the means that the art of man thought proper had been employed for the King's distemper.' Charles himself, maintaining to the last his dry sense of humour, apologised to the crowd assembled in his bedchamber, awaiting the end, that he was taking 'such an unconscionable time a-dying'.[8]

On Friday, Scarburgh noted in his diary, 'Alas! After an ill-fated night His Serene Majesty's strength seemed exhausted to such a degree that the whole assembly of physicians lost all hope and became despondent.' At dawn, Charles asked for the curtains to be opened so that he could see the sunrise and the River Thames one last time, but still they couldn't leave him to die in peace. They bled him again and, now desperate, administered 'an antidote which contained extracts of all the herbs and animals of the kingdom'. They had exhausted the entire apothecary's arsenal and poor Charles too. He could no longer raise his head nor swallow another draft, but one last medication was poured down his throat anyway. When he became breathless, they bled him again. Shortly after, at about 8.30 a.m., the king lost his powers of speech and drifted into a coma. He died at midday, finally relieved of his physicians' attentions, for, as Scarburgh recorded, 'further treatment was made difficult by the death of the king'.

It is now thought that Charles died of uraemia, a condition caused by imminent kidney failure when toxic levels of nitrogen waste build up in the blood. Symptoms of uraemia include confusion, loss of consciousness, low urine production, dry mouth, fatigue, weakness, pale skin or pallor, bleeding problems, rapid heart rate (tachycardia), oedema (swelling) and excessive thirst. It is also painful. When combined with the medical treatments administered – many of which would have exacerbated the symptoms of the illness itself – it shows that the king must have had an incredibly strong constitution to survive for so many days under such an onslaught. As it was said at the time, he died of 'a surfeit of physicians'. It is certainly possible that the medications contributed to or even caused the kidney failure so, if only Charles had been a poor man unable to afford numerous doctors, he may well have recovered from the slight stroke that began his course of treatment.

CONCLUSION

Clearly, medicine has advanced since our ancestors first took up the struggle to overcome disease; our extended life expectancy proves that, even though that is partly down to improvements in diet, sanitation and health and safety as much as any medical breakthroughs. The Royal College of Physicians' concern for public health and preventive medicine has been in evidence since its earliest days. A report on the hazards of industrial work was published in 1627 and another on the dangers of excessive gin drinking in 1726. The college opened the first public dispensary in England in 1698, providing medicine free of charge to the poor, although this move was controversial among its own members.

Advances in antibiotics, antiseptics and anaesthetics have made a dramatic difference to the survival rates of mankind, but I use the word 'advances' deliberately because such things were known to and used by medieval doctors, even without any basic knowledge as to why they worked, giving the patient a better chance of recovery. Lacking such underlying foundations, physicians, surgeons and apothecaries were groping in the dark, often relying on ancient texts that had no more understanding of how the human body worked than they did. Yet little by little, often faced by almost insurmountable opposition, progress was being made.

Sometimes, it was a case of two steps forward and one step back, as in the treatment regimen for the unfortunate Charles II. Recipes for the anaesthetic potion 'dwale' and the beneficial properties of dragon's blood and willow bark seem to have been lost – although willow bark was rediscovered in 1763 by the Revd Edmund Stone, who wrote to the Royal Society pointing out its anti-inflammatory and antipyretic (fever-reducing) effects.

However, experimentation to acquire first-hand knowledge was becoming an acceptable way of learning at last, although discarding the ancient textbooks of Galen and company was a slow and painful process. The first recorded modern 'clinical trial' was conducted onboard HMS *Salisbury* by the naval surgeon James Lind in 1747. During April and May, the ship cruised in the English Channel with the Channel fleet. Although the ships were never far from land, revictualling was a rare occurrence and scurvy began to appear. Over 400 of the fleet's 4,000 mariners were showing symptoms and most of the *Salisbury*'s regular crew were affected to some extent, with nearly eighty out of 350 men seriously weakened. On 20 May, with the agreement of his captain, Lind took aside twelve men with advanced symptoms of scurvy as similar as he could find. For two weeks they shared a diet of mutton broth and boiled biscuit with sugar. Two had a quart of cider a day, two were given twenty-five drops of elixir of vitriol (watered down sulphuric acid) three times a day, two took two spoonfuls of vinegar three times a day, two were dosed with half a pint of seawater a day, two had to swallow an 'electuary' (a medicinal paste made with honey) three times a day, and the final pair were fed two oranges and one lemon a day. This final pair could only receive their treatment for six days before the fruit ran out but, no matter, on the seventh day they were fit enough for duty. Lind also used a control group of several men who were given a 'pain-killing' paste, laxatives and cough syrup. Their condition didn't improve.[1]

This experiment was one of the first controlled trials in medical history, or in any branch of clinical science. The lucky pair who were fed the oranges and lemons, which, according to Lind, they ate 'greedily', were so well recovered after only a week that one returned to normal duties, although his skin still bore the spots of scurvy that had yet to fade and his gums weren't quite back to normal. His companion followed soon after, being given the task of nursing the rest of the group for the remainder of the trial. Those who had drunk the cider also responded favourably but, at the end of two weeks, were still too weak to return to duty. Lind reported no positive effects from vinegar, seawater or the electuary, although the elixir of vitriol made the men's mouths 'much cleaner and in better condition than the rest', with no improvement of other symptoms. Lind concluded that 'the most sudden and visible good effects were perceived from the use of oranges and lemons ... Oranges and lemons were the most effectual remedies for this distemper of the sea.'

Today, we understand why the citrus fruits cured the scurvy sufferers because we know the disease is caused by a deficiency of vitamin C, but nobody had any idea that vitamins existed in the eighteenth century. A process of trial and error was the only way to advance medical science and advance they did.

In this book I have tried to give just a glimpse of the fascinating story of man's attempts to alleviate the pain and suffering of his fellows, but the truth is that I find it impossible to draw any definite conclusions about the continuing process of developing medicine since its earliest origins in the magic and religious beliefs of Stone Age man.

As I write, volunteers are going to West Africa in ever-increasing numbers to assist those who have contracted Ebola, while others work furiously in laboratories to find more effective treatments and, hopefully, a cure and a preventive vaccine. As the fight continues to beat Ebola and other diseases, it is worth remembering that this is simply the most recent chapter in a huge book charting our noble struggle from the most inauspicious beginnings embedded in superstition and the supernatural to enlightened, clinical medicine – one of our species' most magnificent achievements. There will, no doubt, be further challenges in the future. The story of the attempts to unravel the mysteries of medicine isn't finished yet.

ACKNOWLEDGEMENTS

I have so enjoyed putting this book together but nothing would have come of the idea if it hadn't been for all the help and support supplied so willingly by other people.

At the top of my list of those to be thanked must be my husband Glenn. Without his enthusiastic backup, IT know-how and weeks spent scouring sources for suitable images the book would probably have stalled around chapter 6 and been relegated to a bottom drawer.

My very low standard of Latin would have been another huge stumbling block if not for my far more knowledgeable colleagues on the Richard III Society's Research Committee: Dr 'Tig' Lang and Dr Heather Falvey and their respective fields of expertise on medieval remedies (along with caladrius birds and translations of medicinal charms) and the miracles of Henry VI and general assistance with an archaic language. Thank you so much both of you. My thanks also go to Alex Bennett for the enthusiastic receipt of the manuscript – a welcome boost to morale.

My son Steven told me about some of the new work being carried out in his field of pharmaceutical research on substances that sound positively medieval – lizard saliva and snake venom among others – proving we still have much to learn about Nature's secrets.

Acknowledgements

Pat Patrick has generously allowed us to use images from his stock of photographs and also put us in touch with others who have collections of medieval surgical images – a big thank you to him.

As before, I owe a huge debt to Helen Lewer for her professional proofreading skills, grammatical corrections and timely advice on each chapter as it progressed. Will I ever get it right, the difference between 'that' and 'which'?

Many thanks go to Christian Duck, my editor at Amberley, and to her predecessor, Nicola Gale, who set this project in motion back in the spring. Good luck to her in her new career move. Christian always responds so promptly to my email enquiries – a godsend to a harassed writer.

I must thank my inspiring group of mature students in Gravesend for their input during our History of Medicine course this term. Often unwittingly, they supplied new ideas for me to include in the book or provided little anecdotes to liven up the text.

For the paperback reprint, I want to thank Dr S. J. Lang and Dr G. Francis for their helpful comments which have improved the text.

And finally, a huge thank you goes to all my family for their moral support and understanding of Mum's immersion in all things very old and medical and the most appropriate Christmas gifts of books on the subject. These resulted in a hectic week of reading and last-minute additions to the text, references and bibliography as the New Year deadline was rushing towards me.

NOTES

Introduction

1. http://www.catbehaviorassociates.com/why-do-cats-eat-grass/ [accessed 1 December 2014].

2. http://scienceblog.com/983/elephants-eat-dirt-to-supplement-sodium/#2xxeSrsHsH15MZel.97 [accessed 1 December 2014].

3. Gerald, M. C., *The Drug Book* (Toronto, Canada: Sterling, 2013), p. 16.

4. *Ibid.*, p. 16.

5. http://www.bbc.co.uk/news/health-29604204 [accessed 1 December 2014].

1 Dirt, Disease and Danger

1. Hartshorne, P., 'Mooke, fylthe and other vyle things', *BBC History* (August 2014).

2. Kiple, K. F., *Plague, Pox & Pestilence: Disease in History* (London: George Weidenfeld & Nicolson, 1997 [pbk edition; Orion Publishing, 1999]), p. 8.

3. Pollington, S., *Leechcraft: Early English Charms, Plantlore and Healing* (Ely, Cambs: Anglo-Saxon Books, 2000 [2011 edition]), p. 389.

4. Dobson, M., *Disease – The Extraordinary Stories Behind History's Deadliest Killers* (Oxford: Quercus, BCS Publishing Ltd., 2007), p. 140.

5. Furuse, Y., Suzuki, A. & H. Oshitani, 'Origin of the measles virus: divergence from rinderpest virus between the 11th and 12th centuries', *Virology Journal* 7(52) (2010), Online: www.virologyj.com/content/7/1/52 [accessed 25 June 2014]

6. Moses, B., *A Tudor Medicine Chest* (Hodder Wayland, 1997), p. 17.

7. Dobson, M., *Disease – The Extraordinary Stories Behind History's Deadliest Killers* (Oxford: Quercus, BCS Publishing Ltd., 2007), p. 19.

8. Kelly, J., 'A Curse on all Our Houses', *BBC History* (October 2004).

9. Bolton, J. L., 'Looking for *Yersinia pestis*' in Clark, L. & Rawcliffe, C. (eds),

The Fifteenth Century XII (Woodbridge, Suffolk: Boydell and Brewer, 2013), p. 25.

10. *Ibid.*, p. 24.

11. *Ibid.*, p. 31.

12. Robert Henryson, *The Testament of Cresseid* (fifteenth century).

13. Rawcliffe, C., *Medicine & Society in Later Medieval England* (Stroud: Alan Sutton Publishing Ltd, 1995), p. 15.

14. Gant, V. & Thwaites G., 'The Sweating Sickness Returns', *Discover Magazine* (June 1997).

15. www.nhs.uk [accessed 7 July 2014].

16. Robert Lindsay of Pitscottie, *The Historie and Chronicles of Scotland, 1436–1565 (c.* 1532–80).

2 Medicine and the Church

1. French, R., *Medicine Before Science* (Cambridge: University Press, 2003), p. 62.

2. http://www.papalencyclicals.net/Councils/ecum12-2.htm# Clerics to dissociate from shedding-blood [accessed 17 July 2014].

3. Robbins, R. (ed.), *Secular Lyrics of the Fourteenth and Fifteenth Centuries* (Oxford, 1952), pp. 95–96.

4. Pollington, S., *Leechcraft: Early English Charms, Plantlore and Healing* (Ely, Cambs: Anglo-Saxon Books, 2000 [2011 edition]), pp. 454–55.

5. Urry, W., *Thomas Becket: His Last Days* (Stroud: Sutton Publishing Ltd, 1999), p. 145.

6. Knox, R. & Leslie, S., *The Miracles of King Henry VI* ... (Cambridge, 1923), pp. 164–67.

7. Mount, T. P., 'A Manuscript for All Seasons – MS.8004 in the Context of Medieval Medicine and the Dissemination of Knowledge' (unpublished MA thesis concerning a 'Medical and Astrological Compendium' both now at the Wellcome Library of the History and Understanding of Medicine, London, 2009), p. 105.

8. Evans, D., *Placebo* (Oxford: University Press, 2004), p. 1.

9. http://www.british-history.ac.uk/report.aspx?compid=38203 [accessed 10 May 2014].

10. http://klaravonassisi.wordpress.com/2009/01/04/the-rood-of-boxley-or-how-a-lie-grows [accessed 18 July 2014].

11. *Zurich Letters* (The Parker Society), p. 606.

12. Reilly, K., *Automata and Mimesis on the Stage of Theatre History* (Palgrave Macmillan, 2011), p. 21.

13. http://www.forgottenbooks.com/readbook_text/Historical_Papers_1000552124/75 [accessed 24 July 2014], p. 71.

14. http://www.newadvent.org/cathen/04403e.htm [accessed 25 July 2014].

15. http://theknightshospitallers.org/ [accessed 25 July 2014].

16. Stones of Rhodes (rhodonite) at http://en.wikipedia.org/wiki/Rhodonite [accessed 20 May 2014].

3 *Adam Knew Everything!*

1. In 1620 James Ussher, Archbishop of Armagh, had time to fill and added up all the number of years in the Bible since Adam begat ... etc., etc. and Methuselah lived for 187 years and begat Lamech, then lived for another 782 years after that – you get the idea – and worked out that God had created the world on Sunday 23 October 4004 BC.

2. French, R., *Medicine Before Science* (Cambridge: University Press, 2003), pp. 34–5.

3. Parker, S., *Kill or Cure: an Illustrated History of Medicine* (London: Dorling Kindersley Ltd., 2013), p. 41.

4. Mooney, L. R., 'A Middle English Verse Compendium of Astrological Medicine', *Medical History* 28 (1984), pp. 411–12. [I have modernised the spelling.]

5. Dobson, M., *Disease* (Oxford: Quercus, BCS Publishing Ltd, 2007), p. 157.

6. The Book of Daniel, chapter 1, verse 15. King James Bible.

7. http://www.fordham.edu/halsall/source/salimbene1.html A Medieval Sourcebook, Salimbene [accessed 18 August 2014].

8. Haskins, C. H., 'The Latin Literature of Sport', *Speculum* 2(3) (July 1927), p. 244.

9. Rawcliffe, C., *Medicine & Society* (Stroud, Alan Sutton Publishing Ltd, 1995), p. 121.

10. Beck, R. T., *The Cutting Edge – Early History of the Surgeons of London* (London: Lund Humphries, 1974), pp. 62 & 66.

11. *Ibid.*, p. 66.

12. *Ibid.*, p. 63.

13. Thomas, A. H. (ed.), *Calendar of Early Mayor's Court Rolls* (Cambridge: University Press, 1924), p. 5.

14. Beck, R. T., *The Cutting Edge – Early History of the Surgeons of London* (London: Lund Humphries, 1974), p. 135.

15. John Dagvile's will: The National Archives PROB 11/6, Wattys register, 2 November 1477.

16. Jones, P. M., 'Argentine, John, physician and college head', *ODNB*, p. 1.

17. Jones, P. M., 'Information and Science' in *Fifteenth-Century Attitudes*, ed. Rosemary Horrox (1994), p. 107.

18. Horrox, R., 'William Hatteclyffe', *ODNB*.

19. *Ibid.*

20. Mustain, J. K., 'A Rural Medical Practitioner in Fifteenth-Century England' from *Bulletin of the History of Medicine* 46 (1972), p. 473.

21. *Ibid.*, p. 474.

22. Boatwright, L., Habberjam, M. & Hammond, P. (eds), *The Logge Register of PCC Wills, 1479–1486* (Richard III Society, 2008), 1, pp. 164–66.

23. Carlin, M., 'Morstede, Thomas, surgeon', *ODNB*, p. 1.

24. Rawcliffe, C., *Medicine & Society* (Stroud: Alan Sutton Publishing Ltd, 1995), p. 107.

25. *Calendar of Patent Rolls, Edward IV 1461–67*, London,1897, pp. 182–83; *Calendar of Patent Rolls, Edward IV, Henry VI, 1467–77*, London, 1900, p. 211; *Calendar of Patent Rolls, Edward IV, Edward V, Richard III, 1476–85*, London, 1901, pp. 102, 166 & 374.

26. William Hobbys's will: The National Archives PROB 11/8, Milles register, 17 October 1488.

27. *Calendar of Patent Rolls, Edward IV, Edward V, Richard III, 1476–85*, p. 374.

28. John Dagvile's will: The National Archives PROB 11/6, Wattys register, 2 November 1477.

29. Beck, R. T., *The Cutting Edge – Early History of the Surgeons of London* (London: Lund Humphries, 1974), p. 142.

30. Siraisi, N., *Medieval & Early Renaissance Medicine* (London & Chicago: University of Chicago Press, 1990), p. 90.

31. Guildhall Library, London, Guildhall MS.9171/6, 'Wilde', f.192v.

32. Falvey, H., Boatwright, L. & Hammond, P. (editors), *English Wills proved in the Perogative Court of York 1477–99* (Richard III Society, 2013), p. 96.

33. Matthews, L. G., *The Royal Apothecaries* (London: The Wellcome Historical Medical Library, 1967), p. 50.

34. Boatwright, L., Habberjam, M. & Hammond, P. (editors), *The Logge Register of PCC Wills, 1479–1486* (Richard III Society, 2008), vol. 1, pp. 274–76.

35. Dawson, I., *Medicine in the Middle Ages* (London: Hodder Headline Ltd, 2005), p. 37.

36. Matthews, L. G., *The Royal Apothecaries* (London: The Wellcome Historical Medical Library, 1967), p. 11.

4 Diagnosing the Problem

1. Dobson, M., *Disease* (Oxford: Quercus, BCS Publishing Ltd, 2007), p. 244.

2. http://www.diabetes.co.uk/diabetes-history.html [accessed 29 August 2014].

3. http://en.wikipedia.org/wiki/History_of_diabetes [accessed 29 August 2014].

4. MS 8004, 'A Medical and Astrological Compendium' at the Wellcome Library of the History and Understanding of Medicine, London, 1454, f.60v; p. 117.

5. http://www.teagleoptometry.com/history.htm [accessed 7 September 2014].

6. http://courseweb.stthomas.edu/medieval/images/1.4-main.swf [accessed 7 September 2014].

7. http://www.college-optometrists.org/en/college/museyeum/online_exhibitions/spectacles/invention.cfm [accessed 7 September 2014].

8. MS 8004, 'A Medical and Astrological Compendium' at the Wellcome Library of the History and Understanding of Medicine, London, 1454, f.62r.

9. Rawcliffe, C., *Leprosy in Medieval England* (London: Boydell Press, 2009), pp. 186–90.

10. Talbot, C. H., *Medicine in Medieval England* (London: Oldbourne, 1967), p. 131.

11. http://www.greekmedicine.net/diagnosis/Pulse_Diagnosis.html [accessed 8 September 2014].

5 Prognosis – Foretelling Whether the Patient Will Live or Die

1. Parker, S., *Kill or Cure – an Illustrated History of Medicine* (London, New York, etc: Dorling Kindersley Ltd, 2013), pp. 36–37.

2. Rawcliffe, C., *Medicine & Society in Later Medieval England* (Stroud: Alan Sutton Publishing, 1995), p. 87.

3. Egerton MS 2572 at the British Library, ff.50–51.

4. http://archives.wellcomelibrary.org/DServe/dserve.exe?dsqIni=Dserve.ini&dsqApp=Archive&dsqCmd=Show.tcl&dsqDb=Catalog&dsqPos=4&dsqSearch=%28%28%28text%29%3D%27ms%27%29AND%28%28text%29%3D%2740%27%29%29 [accessed 9 November 2014].

5. Campbell, A. M., *The Black Death and Men of Learning* (New York, 1931), pp. 39–42.

6. Page, S., *Astrology in Medieval Manuscripts* (London: The British Library, 2002), p. 16.

7. Rawcliffe, C., *Medicine & Society in Later Medieval England* (Stroud: Alan Sutton Publishing, 1995), p. 86.

8. *Ibid.*, p. 87.

9. Page, S., *Astrology in Medieval Manuscripts* (London: The British Library, 2002), p. 61.

10. Robbins, R., 'Medical Manuscripts in Middle English', *Speculum* 45 (1970), p. 397.

11. MS 8004, 'A Medical and Astrological Compendium' at the Wellcome Library of the History and Understanding of Medicine, London, 1454, ff.65r–67v.

12. *Ibid.*, f.67r.

13. Barber, R., *Bestiary* (Woodbridge: Boydell Press, 1999).

14. *Ibid.*, p. 131.

15. Lang, S., 'The wonderful caladrius bird', *The Ricardian Bulletin* (September 2014), p. 48.

6 Treating the Problem – From the Sensible to the Unbelievable

1. Porter, R. (ed.), *Cambridge Illustrated History of Medicine* (Cambridge: University Press, 1996 [pbk, 2001]), p. 59.

2. Bovey, A., *Tacuinum Sanitatis – An Early Renaissance Guide to Health* (London: Sam Fogg, 2005). My thanks to my MA supervisor at the University of Kent, Dr Alixe Bovey, for this information and a copy of the book.

3. Mount, T. P., 'A Manuscript for All Seasons – MS.8004 in the Context of Medieval Medicine and the Dissemination of Knowledge' (unpublished MA thesis concerning a 'Medical and Astrological Compendium' MS 8004, both now at the Wellcome Library of the History and Understanding of Medicine, London, 2009), pp. 162–64.

4. *Liber Niger Domus Regis*, 1474, Harley MS.642, ff.13–86.

5. http://www.botanical.com/botanical/mgmh/b/betowo35.html [accessed 17 September 2014].

6. Dawson, W. R., *A Leechbook or Collection of Medical Recipes of the Fifteenth Century* (London: Macmillan and Co. Ltd. 1934). The text of MS 136 of the Medical Society of London. Recipe 609, p. 195.

7. http://botanical.com/botanical/mgmh/v/vervai08.html [accessed 17 September 2014].

8. http://botanical.com/botanical/mgmh/m/meadow28.html [accessed 17 September 2014].

9. Nozedar, A., *The Hedgerow Handbook – Recipes, Remedies and Rituals* (London: Random House, Square Peg, 2012), p. 124.

10. Woodward, M. (ed.), *Gerard's Herbal – The History of Plants* (London: Studio Editions, 1994), p. 245.

11. Briggs, D., *A Pinch of Spices* (Essex: Colchester, Blond & Briggs Ltd, 1978), not paginated.

12. Dawson, W. R., *A Leechbook or Collection of Medical Recipes of the Fifteenth Century* (London: Macmillan and Co. Ltd, 1934). The text of MS 136 of the Medical Society of London, Recipe 305, p. 121.

13. *Ibid.*, p. 225.

14. *Ibid.*, p. 319.

15. http://www.thelancet.com/journals/lancet/article/PIIS0140-6736(13)61757-2/fulltext [accessed 20 September 2014].

16. http://botanical.com/botanical/mgmh/w/wormwo37.html [accessed 20 September 2014].

17. http://www.stlukerchamilton.com/Other/StLuke.html [accessed 21 September 2014].

18. Glynn, I. & J., *The Life and Death of Smallpox* (Suffolk: Profile Books Ltd, 2004), p. 26.

19. Wallis F., *Medieval Medicine: a Reader* (Toronto: University Press, 2010), pp. 274–75; http://www.ladydespensersscribery.com/2010/02/22/john-of-gaddesden-smallpox-and-edward-ii/ [accessed 21 September 2014].

20. Finsen, N. R. (trans. J. H. Sequira), *Phototherapy* (London: Arnold, 1901), p. 1.

21. http://www.ncbi.nlm.nih.gov/pubmed/23046014 [accessed 21 September 2014].

22. http://www.discoveriesinmedicine.com/A-An/Antisepsis.html [accessed 22 September 2014].

23. Dawson, W. R., *A Leechbook or Collection of Medical Recipes of the Fifteenth Century* (London: Macmillan and Co. Ltd, 1934). The text of MS 136 of the Medical Society of London, Recipe 356, p. 133.

24. *Ibid.*, p. 263.

25. Parker, S., *Kill or Cure: an Illustrated History of Medicine* (London, New York, etc: Dorling Kindersley Ltd, 2013), p. 52.

26. Williams, B., 'The healing powers of sphagnum moss', *New Scientist* (9 September 1982), pp. 713–14.

27. http://pippap.hubpages.com/hub/Organic-Healing-Treating-Bleeding-Wounds-With-Cobwebs [accessed 28 September 2014].

28. http://www.ncbi.nlm.nih.gov/pmc/articles/PMC3609166/ [accessed 27 September 2014].

29. Dawson, W. R., *A Leechbook or Collection of Medical Recipes of the Fifteenth Century* (London: Macmillan and Co. Ltd, 1934). The text of MS 136 of the Medical Society of London. Recipe 548, p. 177.

30. Both remedies from Moses, B., *A Tudor Medicine Chest* (Great Britain: Hodder Wayland, 1997), p. 15 & p. 21.

31. The *Breviarium Bartholomei* by John Mirfield, British Library, Harley MS. 3.

32. Oxford, Pembroke College, MS 2, f.282.

33. http://www.monarchlabs.com/mdt [accessed 28 September 2014].

34. I want to thank Steven Mount at Astra-Zeneca Laboratories, Macclesfield, for pointing out this new research to me.

35. http://www.economist.com/news/science-and-technology/21569015-snake-venom-being-used-cure-rather-kill-toxic-medicine (5 January 2013) [accessed 29 September 2014].

36. Green, M. H., *The Trotula – An English Translation of the Medieval Compendium of Women's Medicine* (Philadelphia, USA: University of Pennsylvania Press, 2002), p. 70.

37. http://www.ejderhakani.com/infodraga.pdf [accessed 27 September 2014].

38. http://www.worldwidewounds.com/2013/July/Thomas/slug-steve-thomas.html [accessed 10 October 2014].

39. Genesis chapter 30, verses 14–17.

40. Gerald, M. C., *The Drug Book* (New York: Sterling, 2013), p. 34.

41. Green, M. H., *The Trotula – An English Translation of the Medieval Compendium of Women's Medicine* (Philadelphia, USA: University of Pennsylvania Press, 2002), p. 75.

42. *Ibid.*, p. 130.

43. *Ibid.*, pp. 130–31.

44. Pickover, C. A., *The Medical Book – from Witch Doctors to Robot Surgeons, 250 Milestones in the History of Medicine* (New York: Sterling Publishing, 2012), p. 44.

45. Laws, B., *Fifty Plants that Changed the Course of History* (Hove, Kent: Quid Publishing, 2012), p. 217.

46. Wallis F., *Medieval Medicine: a Reader* (Toronto: University Press, 2010), pp. 176–77.

7 *When the Doctor – or the Patient – Is a Woman*

1. http://www.huffingtonpost.com/2012/08/19/todd-akin-abortion-legitimate-rape_n_1807381.html [accessed 4 October 2014].

2. http://www.wondersandmarvels.com/2012/10/two-medieval-women-physicians-tracy-barrett.html [accessed 20 September 2014].

3. Green, M. H., *The Trotula – An English Translation of the Medieval Compendium of Women's Medicine* (Philadelphia, USA: University of Pennsylvania Press, 2002), pp. 76–77.

4. *Ibid.*, p. 77.

5. Parker, S., *Kill or Cure: an Illustrated History of Medicine* (London, New York etc: Dorling Kindersley Ltd., 2013), p. 166.

6. Green, M. H., *The Trotula – An English Translation of the Medieval Compendium of Women's Medicine* (Philadelphia, USA: University of Pennsylvania Press, 2002), p. 79.

7. *Ibid.*, p. 82.

8. *Ibid.*, p. 82.

9. *Ibid.*, p. 78.

10. *Ibid.*, p. 68.

11. Brewer, C., *The Death of Kings – A Medical History of the Kings and Queens of England* (London: Abson Books, 2000), p. 109–10.

12. Green, M. H., *The Trotula – An English Translation of the Medieval Compendium of Women's Medicine* (Philadelphia, USA: University of Pennsylvania Press, 2002), pp. 114–122.

13. Parker, S., *Kill or Cure: an Illustrated History of Medicine* (London, New York etc: Dorling Kindersley Ltd., 2013), p. 167.

14. Wyman, A. L., 'The surgeoness: the female practitioner of surgery 1400–1800' in *Medical History* (1984), 28, pp. 22–41, p. 34.

15. *Ibid.*, p. 28.

16. *Ibid.*, p. 26.

17. Beck, R. T., *The Cutting Edge – Early History of the Surgeons of London* (London: Lund Humphries Publishers Ltd, 1974), p. 75.

18. http://rosaliegilbert.com/births.html [accessed 18 September 2014].

19. *Ibid.*

20. Lang, S. J., the Richard III Society website, 2006.

21. Austin, T. (ed.), *Two Fifteenth-Century Cookery-Books: about 1430–1450* (London: Early English Text Society, 1888), pp. 106–07.

22. My thanks to Dr S. J. Lang for this quotation and access to her extensive work on medicine among the women of the Paston family household.

8 Malpractice and Misbehaviour – Medicine Goes to Court

1. Rawcliffe, C., *Medicine & Society in Later Medieval England* (Stroud: Alan Sutton Publishing Ltd, 1995), p. 111.

2. *Ibid.*, p. 110.

3. Talbot, C. H. & Hammond, E. A., *The Medical Practitioners in Medieval England – A Biographical Register* (London: Wellcome Historical Medical Library, 1965), p. 417.

4. Rawcliffe, C., *Medicine & Society in Later Medieval England* (Stroud: Alan Sutton Publishing Ltd, 1995), p. 12–14.

5. Coghill, N. (ed.), *Geoffrey Chaucer – The Canterbury Tales* (Penguin Books, 1977), p. 31.

6. Chaucer, G., *The Romaunt of the Rose,* Fragment B, lines 5733–38, transcribed into modern English by the author.

7. Voigts, L. E., 'Nicholas Colnet', *ODNB*.

8. Talbot, C. H. & Hammond, E. A., *The Medical Practitioners in Medieval England – A Biographical Register* (London: Wellcome Historical Medical Library, 1965), pp. 369–70.

9. *Ibid.*, p. 164.

10. http://www.bl.uk/manuscripts/Viewer.aspx?ref=harley_ms_1735_fo36v–f.37v.

11. Talbot, C. H., *Medicine in Medieval England* (London: Oldbourne, 1967), p. 137.

12. Talbot, C. H. & Hammond, E. A., *The Medical Practitioners in Medieval England – A Biographical Register* (London: Wellcome Historical Medical Library, 1965), p. 137.

13. *Calendar of Pleas and Memoranda Rolls of the City of London, 1413–1437* (Cambridge: University Press, 1943), pp. 174–75.

14. Cosman, M. P., 'Medieval Medical Malpractice', *The Bulletin of the New York Academy of Medicine* 49(1) (January 1973), p. 27.

15. Ussery, H. E., *Chaucer's Physician – Medicine and Literature in Fourteenth-Century England* (Tulane University, 1971), pp. 27–28.

16. Cosman, M. P., 'Medieval Medical Malpractice' in *The Bulletin of the New York Academy of Medicine* 49(1) (January 1973), pp. 22–47.

17. *Ibid.*, p. 29.

18. Getz, F. M., *Medicine in the English Middle Ages* (Princeton University Press, 1998), p. 79.

19. Talbot, C. H. & Hammond, E. A., *The Medical Practitioners in Medieval England – A Biographical Register* (London: Wellcome Historical Medical Library, 1965), p. 241.

20. McSheffrey, S., *Marriage, Sex and Civic Culture in Late Medieval London* (Philadelphia: University of Pennsylvania Press, 2006), p. 170.

21. *Ibid.*, note 9, p. 251.

22. Castor, H., BBC TV, *Medieval Lives: Birth, Marriage, Death – A Good Marriage* (screened on BBC 4, 16 October 2013) and McSheffrey, S., *Marriage, Sex and Civic Culture in Late Medieval London* (Philadelphia: University of Pennsylvania Press, 2006), pp. 166–76.

23. PROB 11/8 William Hobbys, 'Milles', 17 October 1488, William Hobby's will, National Archives online [accessed January 2005] & translated & transcribed by the author in Mount, T., *The Professionalisation of Medicine in the Fifteenth Century* (Open University BA Honours thesis, 2005).

24. http://en.wikipedia.org/wiki/Derek_Derenalagi [accessed 19 October 2014].

25. http://www.denverpost.com/breakingnews/ci_25340662/mississippi-man-who-woke-up-body-bag-dies [accessed 19 October 2014].

26. My thanks to 'G.P. Sue' on the Open University Advanced Creative Writing Forum in 2011 for this information.

27. Goldberg, P. J. P. (trans. & ed.), *Women in England c. 1275–1525* (Manchester: University Press, 1995), pp. 219–22.

28. *Ibid.*, pp. 119–20.

29. Griffiths, R. A. & Thomas, R. S., *The Making of the Tudor Dynasty* (Gloucester: Alan Sutton Publishing, 1985 [pbk edition, 1987]), pp. 91–93.

9 *Medicine on the Battlefield*

1. Lamont-Brown, R., *Royal Poxes & Potions – The Lives of Court Physicians, Surgeons & Apothecaries* (Stroud: Sutton Publishing, 2001), p. 15.

2. Brewer, C., *The Death of Kings – A Medical History of the Kings and Queens of England* (London: Abson Books, 2000), p. 43.

3. Rosenman, L. D. (ed. and trans.), *The Chirurgia of Roger Frugard* (Xlibris Corporation, 2002), p. 47.

4. Goodman, K., *Ouch! A History of Arrow Wound Treatment* (Dudley: Bows, Blades and Battles Press, 2012), p. 73.

5. http://www.dailymail.co.uk/news/article-2149710/Richard-Lionhearts-death-investigated-French-forensic-scientist--812-years-infection-killed-him.html #ixzz3GgQqUrJe [accessed 20 October 2014].

6. http://motherboard.vice.com/en_uk/blog/scientists-analyze-the-long-dead-heart-of-richard-the-lionheart [accessed 20 October 2014].

7. MS Harley 1736, f.48, (British Library) – I have modernised the spelling.

8. My thanks go to Dr S. J. Lang for sending me an image of a reconstructed copy of Bradmore's instrument which she commissioned and tested very successfully – on a pig's carcase.

9. Lang, S. J., 'John Bradmore and his Book Philomena' in *Archives and Sources, The Society for the Social History of Medicine*, 1992.

10. Beck, R. T., *The Cutting Edge – The Early History of the Surgeons of London* (London: Lund Humphries, 1974), p. 117.

11. 'The battle of Towton: nasty, brutish and not that short', http://www.economist.com/node/17722650 [accessed 21 October 2014].

12. Miller, H., *Secrets of the Dead* (London & Oxford: Macmillan Publishers Ltd, 2000), pp. 33–34.

13. Fiorato, V. *et al.*, *Blood Red Roses – The Archaeology of a Mass Grave from the Battle of Towton AD 1461* (Oxford: Oxbow Books, 2000), pp. 246–47.

14. 'The Wars of the Roses', *Military History Monthly* 50 (November 2014), p. 36.

15. MS. Stowe 440, 'extracted out of the indentures of military service preserved in the Office of Pells by the industry of Sir William Le Neve, Knt, Clarentius King of Arms', before 1664 in the British Library.

16. Appleby, J. *et al.*, 'Perimortem trauma in King Richard III: a skeletal analysis' in *The Lancet*, http://dx.doi.org/10.1016/ S0140-6736(14)60804-7 [accessed 18 September 2014].

17. *Ibid.*

18. *Ibid.*

19. *Ibid.*

20. *Ibid.*

21. Appleby, J. *et al.*, 'The scoliosis of Richard III, last Plantagenet King of England: diagnosis and clinical significance', *The Lancet* 383(9932) (31 May 2014), p. 1944.

10 Passing on Ideas

1. Parker, S., *Kill or Cure: an Illustrated History of Medicine* (London, New York, etc: Dorling Kindersley Ltd, 2013), pp. 100–02.

2. Skeat, W. W. (ed.), *The Complete Works of Geoffrey Chaucer* (Oxford: University Press, 1912 [1946 edition]), p. 424, lines 429–434.

3. http://en.wikipedia.org/wiki/Gilbertus_Anglicus [accessed 1 November 2014].

4. Getz, F. M., *Healing and Society in Medieval England: a Middle English Translation of the Pharmaceutical Writings of Gilbertus Anglicus* (Wisconsin and London, 1991), p. 353.

5. Getz, F. M., 'Gilbertus Anglicus Anglicized' in *Medical History* 26 (1982), p. 441.

6. Lindberg, D. C., *Science in the Middle Ages* (University of Chicago Press, 1978), p. 410.

7. Ziegler, P., *The Black Death* (Cambridgeshire and St Ives: Penguin Books, 1969 [reprinted 1982]), pp. 71–72.

8. *Ibid.*, p. 19.

9. http://biography.yourdictionary.com/guy-de-chauliac [accessed 2 November 2014].

10. http://www.bl.uk/manuscripts/FullDisplay.aspx?ref=Harley_MS_2558 [accessed 3 November 2014].

11. British Library, Harley MS 2558, f. 9.

12. Jones, P. M., 'Thomas Fayreford', *ODNB*.

13. Jones, P. M. 'Thomas Fayreford: An English Fifteenth-Century Medical Practitioner' in French, R. *et al.* (eds), *Medicine from the Black Death to the French Disease* (Aldershot: Ashgate, 1998), p. 173.

14. *Ibid.*, p. 170.

15. *Ibid.*, p. 173.

16. Wallis, F., *Medieval Medicine: a Reader* (Toronto University Press, 2010), p. 314.

17. Mitchell, L., Thomas Fayreford and the transmission of secrets and recipes in Harley MS 2558 (Canada: University of Saskatchewan), http://www.ichstm2013.com/programme/guide/p/1622.html [accessed 3 November 2014].

18. Jones, P. M. 'Thomas Fayreford: An English Fifteenth-Century Medical Practitioner' in French, R. *et al.* (eds), *Medicine from the Black Death to the French Disease* (Aldershot: Ashgate, 1998), p. 168.

19. *Ibid.*, p. 177.

20. Thomas Fayreford's Commonplace Book, digitalised Harley MS 2558, f.125r at: http://www.bl.uk/manuscripts/Viewer.aspx?ref=harley_ms_2558_f125r [accessed 4 November 20 14]. My thanks go to S. J. Lang for correcting my transcription and filling in the blanks with one exception which defeated us both.

21. Jones, P. M., 'Thomas Fayreford', *ODNB*.

22. Jones, P. M., 'Information and Science' in Rosemary Horrox (ed.) *Fifteenth Century Attitudes* (Cambridge: University Press, 1994, pp. 97–111), p. 107.

23. Macdougall, S., 'Health, Diet, Medicine and the Plague' in Chris Given-Wilson (ed.), *An Illustrated History of Late-Medieval England* (Manchester: University Press, 1996), p. 99.

24. Beck, R. T., *The Cutting Edge – Early History of the Surgeons of London* (London: Lund Humphries Publishers Ltd, 1974), p. 109.

25. *Ibid.*, p. 108.

26. *Ibid.*, p. 108.

27. Richard Esty's will: Guildhall Library, London, Guildhall MS.9171/6, 'Wilde', f.192v.

28. Both in Beck, R. T., *The Cutting Edge – Early History of the Surgeons of London* (London: Lund Humphries Publishers Ltd, 1974), p. 163, 166.

29. Rawcliffe, C., *Medicine & Society in Later Medieval England* (Stroud: Alan Sutton Publishing Ltd, 1995), p. 129.

30. http://www.ncbi.nlm.nih.gov/pubmed/17961048 [accessed 3 November 2014].

31. http://en.wikipedia.org/wiki/Guido_da_Vigevano [accessed 3 November 2014].

11 Tudor Medicine

1. Furdell, E. L., 'Andrew Boorde', *ODNB*.

2. http://www.britannica.com/EBchecked/topic/73671/Andrew-Boorde [accessed 28 October 2014].

3. Boorde, A., *Compendyous Regyment or Dyetary of Health*, 1542.

4. *Ibid.*

5. http://en.wikipedia.org/wiki/Paracelsus [accessed 29 October 2014].

6. http://www.sciencemuseum.org.uk/broughttolife/people/paracelsus.asp [accessed 29 October 2014].

7. Dawson, I., *The History of Medicine: Renaissance Medicine* (London: Hodder Wayland, 2005), p. 16.

8. Pickover, C. A., *The Medical Book – from Witch Doctors to Robot Surgeons, 250 Milestones in the History of Medicine* (New York: Sterling Publishing, 2012), p. 70.

9. http://www.sciencemuseum.org.uk/broughttolife/people/paracelsus.asp [accessed 29 October 2014].

10. http://en.wikipedia.org/wiki/Paracelsus [accessed 29 October 2014].

11. Jacobi, J. (ed) & Guterman, N. (trans.), *Paracelsus, Selected Writings* (New York: Pantheon, 1951), p. 79–80.

12. Dawson, I., *The History of Medicine: Renaissance Medicine* (London: Hodder Wayland, 2005), p. 12.

13. Pickover, C. A., *The Medical Book – from Witch Doctors to Robot Surgeons, 250 Milestones in the History of Medicine* (New York: Sterling Publishing, 2012), p. 72.

14. Dawson, I., *The History of Medicine: Renaissance Medicine* (London: Hodder Wayland, 2005), p. 15.

15. *Ibid.*, p. 18.

16. http://www.britannica.com/EBchecked/topic/336408/Leonardo-da-Vinci/59785/Anatomical-studies-and-drawings [accessed 4 November 2014].

17. http://embryo.asu.edu/pages/leonardo-da-vincis-embryological-drawings-fetus#sthash [accessed 1 November 2014].

18. Bodleian Laud Miscellaneous MS 724, f.97r at: http://bodley30.bodley.ox.ac.uk:8180/luna/servlet/view/all/who/Albucasis%20(Abu%20al-Qasim%20Khalaf%20ibn%20'Abbas%20al-Zahrawi)/what/MS.%20Laud%20Misc.%20724?os=0&pgs=50 [accessed 1 November 2014].

19. http://www.livescience.com/20157-anatomy-drawings-leonardo-da-vinci.html [accessed 4 November 2014].

20. https://www.rcplondon.ac.uk/about/history [accessed 29 October 2014].

21. *Ibid.*

22. http://www.nndb.com/people/759/000082513/ [accessed 30 October 2014].

23. Brewer, C., *The Death of Kings – A Medical History of the Kings and Queens of England* (London: Abson Books, 2000), p. 123.

24. http://www.historyextra.com/feature/tudors/5-things-you-probably-didn%E2%80%99t-know-about-henry-viii [accessed 30 October 2014].

25. Lamont-Brown, R., *Royal Poxes & Potions – The Lives of Court Physicians, Surgeons & Apothecaries* (Gloucester: Sutton Publishing, 2001), p. 33.

26. *Ibid.*, p. 33.

27. My thanks go to Helen Lewer for pointing out that this problem is known as Cushing's disease.

28. Brewer, C., *The Death of Kings – A Medical History of the Kings and Queens of England* (London: Abson Books, 2000), pp. 123–24.

29. Lamont-Brown, R., *Royal Poxes & Potions – The Lives of Court Physicians, Surgeons & Apothecaries* (Gloucester: Sutton Publishing, 2001), p. 33.

30. Brewer, C., *The Death of Kings – A Medical History of the Kings and Queens of England* (London: Abson Books, 2000), p. 128.

31. *Ibid.*, p. 128.

32. *Ibid.*, p. 136.

33. *Ibid.*, p. 146.

34. http://news.bbc.co.uk/1/hi/magazine/5159022.stm [accessed 31 October 2014].

35. Lamont-Brown, R., *Royal Poxes & Potions – The Lives of Court Physicians, Surgeons & Apothecaries* (Gloucester: Sutton Publishing, 2001), pp. 35–36.

36. http://www.elizabethan-era.org.uk/death-of-queen-elizabeth-i.htm [accessed 29 October 2014].

37. http://www.yourdentistryguide.com/tooth-abscess/ [accessed 31 October 2014].

38. Elmer, P & Grell, O. P. (eds), *Health, Disease and Society in Europe, 1500–1800 – a source book* (Manchester University Press, in association with the Open University, 2004), p. 257.

39. http://www.sciencemuseum.org.uk/broughttolife/people/ambroisepare.aspx [accessed 30 October 2014].

40. http://en.wikipedia.org/wiki/Ambroise_Par%C3%A9 [accessed 30 October 2014].

41. Elmer, P & Grell, O. P. (eds), *Health, Disease and Society in Europe, 1500–1800 – a source book* (Manchester University Press, in association with the Open University, 2004), p. 258.

42. *Ibid.*, pp. 258–59.

12 *Progress in Medicine?*

1. Bishop, W. J., *Knife, Fire and Boiling Oil* (London: Robert Hale, 2010), pp. 65–66.

2. Roberts, G., *The Mirror of Alchemy – Alchemical Ideas and Images in Manuscripts and Books from Antiquity to the Seventeenth Century* (London: British Library, 1994), p. 55.

3. http://special.lib.gla.ac.uk/exhibns/month/june2007.html (*De Motu Cordis*) [accessed 16 November 2014].

4. http://chelseaphysicgarden.co.uk/the-garden/plant-collections/the-pharmaceutical-garden/ [accessed 10 November 2014].

5. http://cdnmedhall.org/dr-robert-laing-noble [accessed 10 November 2014].

6. http://www.livingrainforest.org/about-rainforests/anti-cancer-rosy-periwinkle/ [accessed 10 November 2014].

7. The Apothecary at St Thomas, http://www.thegarret.org.uk/apothecaries.htm [accessed 8 November 2014].

8. http://www.englishmonarchs.co.uk/stuart_3.htm [accessed 11 November 2014].

Conclusion

1. Harvie, D. I., *Limeys* (Stroud: Sutton Publishing, 2002), pp. 90–91.

BIBLIOGRAPHY

Original sources
'A Medical and Astrological Compendium', Wellcome Library MS 8004
Almanac or Girdle-book, Wellcome Library MS 40
Boorde, Andrew, *Compendyous Regyment or Dyetary of Health* (1542)
Caius, John, *A Boke or Counseill Against the Disease Commonly Called the Sweate, or Sweatyng Sicknesse*
Calendar of Pleas and Memoranda Rolls of the City of London, 1413–1437 (Cambridge University Press, 1943)
Chaucer, Geoffrey, *The Romaunt of the Rose*, Fragment B
Crophill, John, *Commonplace Book*, Harley MS 1735
Fayreford, Thomas, *Commonplace Book*, Harley MS 2558
Guild Book of the Barber Surgeons of York, Egerton MS 2572
Harvey, William, *De Moto Cordis*
Henryson, Robert, *The Testament of Cresseid*
John Dagvile's will, National Archives PROB 11/6, Wattys register, 2 November 1477
Liber Niger Domus Regis, Harley MS 642, ff. 13–86
Richard Esty's will, Guildhall Library MS 9171/6, 'Wilde', f. 192v.
Robert Lindsay of Pitscottie, *The Historie and Chronicles of Scotland, 1436–1565*
The Breviarium Bartholomei, Harley MS 3
William Hobbys's will, National Archives PROB 11/8, Milles register, 17 October 1488, translated & transcribed by the author in Mount, T., *The Professionalisation of Medicine in the Fifteenth Century* (Open University BA Honours thesis, 2005)

Secondary sources

'A Tale for Our Times', Online: http://news.bbc.co.uk/1/hi/magazine/5159022. stm [accessed 31 October 2014]

'Ambroise Paré (1510–90)', Online: http://www.sciencemuseum.org.uk/ broughttolife/people/ambroisepare.aspx [accessed 30 October 2014]

'Anti-cancer: Rosy Periwinkle', Online: http://www.livingrainforest.org/about-rainforests/anti-cancer-rosy-periwinkle/ [accessed 10 November 2014]

'Dr Robert Laing Noble', Online: http://cdnmedhall.org/dr-robert-laing-noble [accessed 10 November 2014]

'Ebola: Is Bushmeat Behind the Outbreak?', Online: http://www.bbc.co.uk/news/ health-29604204 [accessed 1 December 2014]

'Elephants Eat Dirt to Supplement Sodium', Online: http://scienceblog.com/983/ elephants-eat-dirt-to-supplement-sodium/#2xxeSrsHsH15MZel.97 [accessed 1 December 2014]

'Fourth Lateran Council: 1215', Online: www.papalencyclicals.net/Councils/ ecum12-2.htm [accessed 17 July 2014]

'Guy de Chauliac Facts', Online: http://biography.yourdictionary.com/guy-de-chauliac [accessed 2 November 2014]

'History of the RCP', Online: https://www.rcplondon.ac.uk/about/history [accessed 29 October 2014]

'Houses of Cistercian monks: The abbey of Boxley', Online: http://www.british-history.ac.uk/report.aspx?compid=38203 [accessed 10 May 2014]

'John Caius', Online: http://www.nndb.com/people/759/000082513/ [accessed 30 October 2014]

'John of Gaddesden, Smallpox and Edward II', Online: http://www. ladydespensersscribery.com/2010/02/22/john-of-gaddesden-smallpox-and-edward-ii/ [accessed 21 September 2014]

'Knights Hospitallers of the Sovereign Order of St John of Jerusalem Knights of Malta', Online: http://theknightshospitallers.org/ [accessed 25 July 2014]

'Meadowsweet', Online: http://botanical.com/botanical/mgmh/m/meadow28. html [accessed 17 September 2014]

'Medical Maggots', Online: http://www.monarchlabs.com/mdt [accessed 28 September 2014]

'Medieval Births and Birthing', Online: http://rosaliegilbert.com/births.html [accessed 18 September 2014]

'Medieval Sourcebook: Salimbene: On Frederick II, 13th Century', Online: http:// www.fordham.edu/halsall/source/salimbene1.html [accessed 18 August 2014]

'Mississippi Man Who Woke up in a Body Bag Dies', Online: http://www. denverpost.com/breakingnews/ci_25340662/mississippi-man-who-woke-up-body-bag-dies [accessed 19 October 2014]

'Organic Healing: Using Spiders' Webs to Heal', Online: http://pippap.hubpages. com/hub/Organic-Healing-Treating-Bleeding-Wounds-With-Cobwebs [accessed 28 September 2014]

'Pulse Diagnosis', Online: http://www.greekmedicine.net/diagnosis/Pulse_ Diagnosis.html [accessed 8 September 2014]

'Richard the Lionheart's Heart to be Examined ... 812 Years after Mystery Infection Killed Him', *Daily Mail*, Online: http://www.dailymail.co.uk/news/ article-2149710/Richard-Lionhearts-death-investigated-French-forensic- scientist--812-years-infection-killed-him.html#ixzz3GgQqUrJe [accessed 20 October 2014]

'Snake Venom Is Being Used to Cure, Rather than Kill', Online: http://www. economist.com/news/science-and-technology/21569015-snake-venom-being- used-cure-rather-kill-toxic-medicine [accessed 29 September 2014]

'St Luke', Online: http://www.stlukerchamilton.com/Other/StLuke.html [accessed 21 September 2014]

'Sts Cosmas & Damian', Online: http://www.newadvent.org/cathen/04403e.htm [accessed 25 July 2014]

'The battle of Towton: nasty, brutish and not that short', Online: http://www. economist.com/node/17722650 [accessed 21 October 2014]

'The House of Stuart: Charles II', Online: http://www.englishmonarchs.co.uk/ stuart_3.htm [accessed 11 November 2014]

'The Neuroanatomical Plates of Guido da Vigevano', Online: http://www.ncbi. nlm.nih.gov/pubmed/17961048 [accessed 3 November 2014]

'The Pharmaceutical Garden', Online: http://chelseaphysicgarden.co.uk/ the-garden/plant-collections/the-pharmaceutical-garden/ [accessed 10 November 2014]

'The Rood of Boxley; or, How a lie grows', Online: http://klaravonassisi. wordpress.com/2009/01/04/the-rood-of-boxley-or-how-a-lie-grows [accessed 18 July 2014]

'Tooth Abscess: Causes, Symptoms and Treatment of Abscesses', Online: http:// www.yourdentistryguide.com/tooth-abscess/ [accessed 31 October 2014]

'Vervain', Online: http://botanical.com/botanical/mgmh/v/vervai08.html [accessed 17 September 2014]

'Why Do Cats Eat Grass?', Online: http://www.catbehaviorassociates.com/ why-do-cats-eat-grass/ [accessed 1 December 2014]

'Wormwoods', Online: http://botanical.com/botanical/mgmh/w/wormwo37.html [accessed 20 September 2014]

Appleby, J. *et al.*, 'Perimortem trauma in King Richard III: a skeletal analysis' in *The Lancet*, Online: http://dx.doi.org/10.1016/ S0140-6736(14)60804-7 [accessed 18 September 2014]

Barber, R., *Bestiary* (Woodbridge: Boydell Press, 1999)

Beck, R. T., *The Cutting Edge – The Early History of the Surgeons of London* (London: Lund Humphries, 1974)

Bishop, W. J., *Knife, Fire and Burning Oil – The Early History of Surgery* (London: Robert Hale, 2010)

Boatwright, L., Habberjam, M. & Hammond, P. (eds), *The Logge Register of PCC Wills, 1479–1486* (Richard III Society, 2008)

Bolton, J. L., 'Looking for *Yersinia pestis*' in Clark, L & Rawcliffe, C. (eds), *The Fifteenth Century XII* (Woodbridge: Boydell and Brewer, 2013)

Bovey, A., *Tacuinum Sanitatis – An Early Renaissance Guide to Health* (London: Sam Fogg, 2005)

Brewer, C., *The Death of Kings – A Medical History of the Kings and Queens of England* (London: Abson Books, 2000)

Briggs, D., *A Pinch of Spices* (Colchester: Blond & Briggs Ltd, 1978)

Campbell, A. M., *The Black Death and Men of Learning* (New York: 1931)

Coghill, N. (ed.), *Geoffrey Chaucer – The Canterbury Tales* (Penguin Books, 1977)

Considine, A., Richard the Lionheart Wasn't Poisoned, Analysis of the Long-Dead King's Heart Shows', Online: http://motherboard.vice.com/en_uk/blog/scientists-analyze-the-long-dead-heart-of-richard-the-lionheart [accessed 20 October 2014]

Cosman, M. P., 'Medieval Medical Malpractice', *The Bulletin of the New York Academy of Medicine* 49(1) (January 1973), pp. 22–47

Dawson, I., *The History of Medicine: Renaissance Medicine* (London: Hodder Wayland, 2005)

Dawson, W. R., *A Leechbook or Collection of Medical Recipes of the Fifteenth Century* (London: Macmillan and Co. Ltd, 1934)

Dobson, M., *Disease – The Extraordinary Stories Behind History's Deadliest Killers* (Oxford: Quercus, BCS Publishing Ltd, 2007)

Drewry, R. D., 'What Man Devised That He Might See', Online: http://www.teagleoptometry.com/history.htm [accessed 7 September 2014]

Elmer, P & Grell, O. P. (eds), *Health, Disease and Society in Europe, 1500–1800 – a source book* (Manchester University Press, in association with the Open University, 2004)

Evans, D., *Placebo* (Oxford: University Press, 2004)

Falvey, H., Boatwright, L. & Hammond, P. (eds), *English Wills proved in the Perogative Court of York 1477–99* (Richard III Society, 2013)

Finsen, N. R. (trans. J. H. Sequira), *Phototherapy* (London: Arnold, 1901)

Fiorato, V. *et al.*, *Blood Red Roses – The Archaeology of a Mass Grave from the Battle of 'Towton AD 1461* (Oxford: Oxbow Books, 2000)

French, R., *Medicine Before Science* (Cambridge: University Press, 2003)

Furdell, E. L., 'Andrew Boorde', *ODNB*

Furuse, Y., Suzuki, A. & H. Oshitani, 'Origin of the measles virus: divergence from rinderpest virus between the 11th and 12th centuries', *Virology Journal* 7(52) (2010), Online: www.virologyj.com/content/7/1/52 [accessed 25 June 2014]

Gant, V. & Thwaites, G., 'The Sweating Sickness Returns', *Discover Magazine* (June 1997)

Gerald, M. C., *The Drug Book* (New York: Sterling, 2013)

Getz, F. M., 'Gilbertus Anglicus Anglicized', *Medical History* 26 (1982)

Getz, F. M., *Healing and Society in Medieval England: a Middle English Translation of the Pharmaceutical Writings of Gilbertus Anglicus* (Wisconsin & London, 1991)

Getz, F. M., *Medicine in the English Middle Ages* (Princeton University Press, 1998)

Glynn, I. & J., *The Life and Death of Smallpox* (Suffolk: Profile Books Ltd, 2004)

Goldberg, P. J. P. (ed. and trans.) *Women in England c. 1275–1525* (Manchester: University Press, 1995)

Goodman, K., *Ouch! A History of Arrow Wound Treatment* (Dudley: Bows, Blades and Battles Press, 2012)

Green, M. H., *The Trotula – An English Translation of the Medieval Compendium of Women's Medicine* (University of Pennsylvania Press, 2002)

Griffiths, R. A. & Thomas, R. S., *The Making of the Tudor Dynasty* (Gloucester: Alan Sutton Publishing Ltd, 1985 [pbk edition, 1987])

Hartshorne, P., 'Mooke, fylthe and other vyle things', *BBC History* (August 2014)

Harvie, D. I., *Limeys* (Stroud: Sutton Publishing, 2002)

Haskins, C. H., 'The Latin Literature of Sport', *Speculum* 2(3) (July 1927), p. 244.

Heydenreich, L. H., 'Leonardo da Vinci: Anatomical Studies and Drawings', Online: http://www.britannica.com/EBchecked/topic/336408/Leonardo-da-Vinci/59785/Anatomical-studies-and-drawings [accessed 4 November 2014]

Hong, J. S., Jung, J. Y., Yoon, J. Y. & D. H. Suh, 'Acne treatment by methyl aminolevulinate photodynamic therapy with red light vs. intense pulsed light', Online: http://www.ncbi.nlm.nih.gov/pubmed/23046014 [accessed 21 September 2014]

Horrox, R. (ed.), *Fifteenth Century Attitudes* (Cambridge: University Press, 1994)

Horrox, R., 'William Hatteclyffe', *ODNB*

Jacobi, J. (ed.) & Guterman, N. (trans.), *Paracelsus, Selected Writings* (New York: Pantheon, 1951)

Jones, P. M., 'Thomas Fayreford: An English Fifteenth-Century Medical

Practitioner', in French, R. *et al.* (eds), *Medicine from the Black Death to the French Disease* (Aldershot: Ashgate, 1998), pp. 156–81.

Jones, P. M., 'Thomas Fayreford', *ODNB*

Kelly, J., 'A Curse on all Our Houses', *BBC History* (October 2004)

Kiple, K. F., *Plague, Pox & Pestilence: Disease in History* (London: George Weidenfeld & Nicolson, 1997 [pbk edition Orion Publishing, 1999])

Knox, R. & Leslie, S., *The Miracles of King Henry VI: being an account and translation of twenty-three miracles taken from the manuscript in the British Library, Royal 13c.viii...* (Cambridge, 1923)

Lamont-Brown, R., *Royal Poxes & Potions – The Lives of Court Physicians, Surgeons & Apothecaries* (Gloucester: Sutton Publishing, 2001)

Lang, S. J., 'John Bradmore and his Book Philomena', *Social History of Medicine* 5 (1992)

Lang, S. J., 'The wonderful caladrius bird', *The Ricardian Bulletin* (September 2014)

Laws, B., *Fifty Plants that Changed the Course of History* (Hove: Quid Publishing, 2012)

Lindberg, D. C., *Science in the Middle Ages* (University of Chicago Press, 1978)

Macdougall, S., 'Health, Diet, Medicine and the Plague' in C. Given-Wilson (ed.), *An Illustrated History of Late-Medieval England* (Manchester: University Press, 1996)

Matthews, L. G., *The Royal Apothecaries* (London: The Wellcome Historical Medical Library, 1967)

McFarnon, E., '5 Things You (Probably) Didn't Know about Henry VIII', Online: http://www.historyextra.com/feature/tudors/5-things-you-probably-didn%E2%80%99t-know-about-henry-viii [accessed 30 October 2014]

McSheffrey, S., *Marriage, Sex and Civic Culture in Late Medieval London* (University of Pennsylvania Press, 2006)

Miller, H., *Secrets of the Dead* (London & Oxford: Macmillan Publishers Ltd, Channel 4 Books, 2000)

Mitchell, L., 'Thomas Fayreford and the transmission of secrets and recipes in Harley MS 2558' (Canada: University of Saskatchewan), Online: http://www.ichstm2013.com/programme/guide/p/1622.html [accessed 3 November 2014]

Mitchell, P. D., Hui-Yuan, Y., Appleby, J. & R. Buckley, 'The Intestinal Parasites of King Richard III', Online: http://www.thelancet.com/journals/lancet/article/PIIS0140-6736(13)61757-2/fulltext [accessed 20 September 2014]

Mooney, L. R., 'A Middle English Verse Compendium of Astrological Medicine', *Medical History* 28 (1984)

Morris, J., *Historical Papers* (1893; reprinted London: Forgotten Books, 2013), pp. 70–71

Moses, B., *A Tudor Medicine Chest* (Hodder Wayland, 1997).

Mount, T. P., 'A Manuscript for All Seasons – MS.8004 in the Context of Medieval Medicine and the Dissemination of Knowledge' (unpublished MA thesis concerning a 'Medical and Astrological Compendium' MS 8004, both now at the Wellcome Library of the History and Understanding of Medicine, London, 2009)

Mustain, J. K., 'A Rural Medical Practitioner in Fifteenth-Century England', *Bulletin of the History of Medicine* 46 (1972), p. 473

Nozedar, A., *The Hedgerow Handbook – Recipes, Remedies and Rituals* (London: Random House, Square Peg, 2012)

Page, S., *Astrology in Medieval Manuscripts* (London: The British Library, 2002)

Pappas, S., 'Human Body Part that Stumped Leonardo da Vinci Revealed', Online: http://www.livescience.com/20157-anatomy-drawings-leonardo-da-vinci.html [accessed 4 November 2014]

Parker, S., *Kill or Cure: an Illustrated History of Medicine* (London, New York: Dorling Kindersley Ltd, 2013)

Pickover, C. A., *The Medical Book – from Witch Doctors to Robot Surgeons, 250 Milestones in the History of Medicine* (New York: Sterling Publishing, 2012)

Pollington, S., *Leechcraft: Early English Charms, Plantlore and Healing* (Ely: Anglo-Saxon Books, 2000 [2011 edition])

Porter, R. (ed.), *Cambridge Illustrated History of Medicine* (Cambridge: University Press, 1996 [pbk, 2001])

Rawcliffe, C., *Leprosy in Medieval England* (London: Boydell Press, 2009)

Rawcliffe, C., *Medicine & Society in Later Medieval England* (Stroud: Alan Sutton Publishing Ltd, 1995)

Reilly, K., *Automata and Mimesis on the Stage of Theatre History* (Palgrave Macmillan, 2011)

Reynoldson, F., *Medicine Through Time,* (Oxford: Heinemann, 2001)

Robbins, R. (ed.), *Secular Lyrics of the Fourteenth and Fifteenth Centuries* (Oxford, 1952)

Roberts, G., *The Mirror of Alchemy – Alchemical Ideas and Images in Manuscripts and Books from Antiquity to the Seventeenth Century* (London: British Library, 1994)

Rosenman, L. D. (ed. and trans.), *The Chirurgia of Roger Frugard* (Xlibris Corporation, 2002)

Siraisi, N., *Medieval & Early Renaissance Medicine* (University of Chicago Press, 1990)

Skeat, W. W. (ed.), *The Complete Works of Geoffrey Chaucer* (Oxford: University Press, 1912 [1946 edition])

Talbot, C. H. & Hammond, E. A., *The Medical Practitioners in Medieval*

England – A Biographical Register (London: Wellcome Historical Medical Library, 1965)

Talbot, C. H., *Medicine in Medieval England* (London: Oldbourne, 1967)

Thomas, A. H. (ed.), *Calendar of Early Mayor's Court Rolls* (Cambridge: University Press, 1924)

Thomas, S., 'Medicinal use of terrestrial molluscs (slugs and snails) with particular reference to their role in the treatment of wounds and other skin lesions', Online: http://www.worldwidewounds.com/2013/July/Thomas/slug-steve-thomas.html [accessed 10 October 2014]

Urry, W., *Thomas Becket: His Last Days* (Stroud: Sutton Publishing, 1999)

Ussery, H. E., *Chaucer's Physician – Medicine and Literature in Fourteenth-Century England* (Louisiana: Tulane University, 1971)

Voigts, L. E., 'Nicholas Colnet' *ODNB*

Wallis F., *Medieval Medicine: a Reader* (Toronto: University Press, 2010)

Williams, B., 'The healing powers of sphagnum moss', *New Scientist* (9 September 1982), pp. 713–14

Woodward, M. (ed.), *Gerard's Herbal – The History of Plants* (London: Studio Editions, 1994)

Wyman, A. L., 'The surgeoness: the female practitioner of surgery 1400–1800', *Medical History* 28 (1984), pp. 22–41.

Ziegler, P., *The Black Death* (Cambridgeshire and St Ives: Penguin Books, 1969 [reprinted 1982])

LIST OF ILLUSTRATIONS

1. Vespasian suffering from leprosy and being examined in bed by two doctors. British Library, Add 89066 1, f.61v. Eustache Marcadé, *Mystère de la Vengeance de Nostre Seigneur Ihesu Crist*. Burgundy France, 1465. (Courtesy of the British Library)

2. Leper with bell. BL Lansdowne 451. Pontifical Tabular, England, early fifteenth century. (Courtesy of the British Library)

3. Patient with saints Cosmas and Damian. BL Royal 15 E II f.77v. Bartholomaeus Anglicus, *De proprietatibus rerum*, Bruges, 1482. (Courtesy of the British Library)

4. Abbot of Saint Denis consulting a wise-woman. BL Royal 20 C VII f.12 Philip III Chroniques de France ou de St Denis. France, about 1300. (Courtesy of the British Library)

5. Stones of Rhodes and snake stones. (Courtesy of Glenn Mount)

6. Adam naming the animals. Northumberland Bestiary, England, about 1250. (Courtesy of Getty Open Content)

7. First illustration of spectacles. Cardinal Hugh of Saint Claire (Hugh de Provence). Fresco by Tomaso of Modena, Italy, 1352. (Author's collection)

7a. Monks wearing spectacles. Archeon Living History Museum, Netherlands. (Courtesy Hans Splinter)

8. The Four Humours. BL Egerton 2572 f.51v. Calendar, diagrams; medical texts Guild Book of the Barber Surgeons of York, England, about 1486. (Courtesy of the British Library)

9. Urine colour chart. Wellcome Library, London, M0007286. *Epiphaniae medicorum* by Ulrich Pinder, Nuremberg Germany, about 1510. (Courtesy of the Wellcome Library)

10. Vein Man. Wellcome Library, London MS.40 L0020781. Folding Almanac, England, late fifteenth century. (Courtesy of the Wellcome Library)

11. Zodiac man and a volvelle (incomplete). BL Egerton 2572 ff.50v-51. Calendar, diagrams; medical texts. Guild Book of the Barber Surgeons of York, England about 1486. (Courtesy of the British Library)

11a. Reproduction volvelle. (Courtesy of Glenn Mount)

12. Female surgeon cupping a female patient. BL Sloane 6 f.177v. Medical Treatise by John of Arderne, England, mid-fifteenth century. (Courtesy of the British Library)

13. Zodiac Man. BL Sloane 2250, f12. (The man's pointing finger serves as a warning against the powerful forces of the stars astrology.) Physician's folding calendar, England, early fifteenth century. (Courtesy of the British Library)

14. Caladrius bird in action. BL Royal 15 E VI, f.21v. The Talbot Shrewsbury Book, France, 1145. (Courtesy of the British Library)

15. Chenies Manor, Amersham, Buckinghamshire, showing its windowless face to the miasmas of London. (Author's collection)

16. Dragon's blood tree (*Dracaena draco*) in Tenerife. (Courtesy of Esculapio)

16a. Dragon's blood resin. (Courtesy of Andy Dingley)

17. Spheres of Pythagoras. Wellcome Library, London, MS8004 pp. 33, 34. A Physician's Handbook, England, about 1454. (Courtesy of the Wellcome Library)

18. Elephant and a dragon. BL Harley 3244, f.39v. A bestiary, England, about 1250. (Courtesy of the British Library)

19. Mandrake. US National Library of Medicine, Jacob Meydenbach's *Hortus Sanitatis* (Garden of Health) Germany, 1491. (Courtesy of the US National Library of Medicine)

20. Dame Trotula, Empress among midwives. Wellcome Library, London WMS 544 f.65r. France, early fourteenth century. (Courtesy of the Wellcome Library)

21. Jar for Mithridate and Theriac. Getty Open Content, Italian, about 1580. (Courtesy of Getty Open Content)

22. Birth of Caesar by caesarean section. BL Royal 16 G VII f.219, France late fourteenth century. (Courtesy of the British Library)

23. Pregnant woman with possible positions of the foetus. Wellcome Library, London WMS 49 f.38r. *The Apocalypse of St John*, Germany, 1420. (Courtesy of the Wellcome Library)

24. Female surgeon. BL Sloane 6 f.177v. John Arderne's treatise, England, *c*. 1425. (Courtesy of the British Library)

25. Modern replica of John Bradmore's instrument. (Courtesy of Dr S. J. Lang)

26. Wound Man *c*. 1450. Wellcome Library, London. WMS 290 f.53v. *Anathomia*, England mid-fifteenth century. (Courtesy of the Wellcome Library)

27. Surgeon treating patients with broken or dislocated bones. BL Sloane 1977 f.6. Roger Frugard of Parma, France, early fourteenth century. (Courtesy of the British Library)

INDEX

Index

S